A Quiet Voice

A Quiet Voice

✦

One man's journey from Post Traumatic Stress Disorder through addiction, prison and homelessness to a dignified life and a successful career.

Based on a True Story

Eugene Hairston
as told to Susan Adger

iUniverse, Inc.
New York Lincoln Shanghai

A Quiet Voice

One man's journey from Post Traumatic Stress Disorder through addiction, prison and homelessness to a dignified life and a successful career. Based on a True Story

iUniverse books may be ordered through booksellers or by contacting:

iUniverse
2021 Pine Lake Road, Suite 100
Lincoln, NE 68512
www.iuniverse.com
1-800-Authors (1-800-288-4677)

Because of the dynamic nature of the Internet, any Web addresses or links contained in this book may have changed since publication and may no longer be valid.

The views expressed in this work are solely those of the author and do not necessarily reflect the views of the publisher, and the publisher hereby disclaims any responsibility for them.

ISBN: 978-0-595-46647-4 (pbk)
ISBN: 978-0-595-90942-1 (ebk)

Printed in the United States of America

Contents

Acknowledgements and Dedication

I'd like to thank the following people for their support and encouragement during my recovery and the writing of this book:

- To Patrick M., for listening, guiding, and teaching me

- To Mr. C., for being my mentor and helping me to build confidence in myself

- To my AA Home Group, for acceptance, love, laughs, and guidance

- To William E. Hairston, for being MY father and holding fast to morals and values

- To the love of my life, Cathy C., for her patience, love, and for all the laughter—she never once put me down for not knowing something

- To Susan Adger, who co-authored this book and helped to make a dream come true

The section of the book that deals with Vietnam is dedicated to the men I served with there, those who returned and those who did not. As a PTSD survivor, I have blocked out a lot of the past, but I've honestly reported my best recollection of this very difficult time in my life. However, some events may not be completely accurate. This period of my life has passed. I seek no retribution.

Author's Note

This book is based on a true story but some situations may be portrayed differently from what actually took place, either because I cannot remember exactly the sequence of events, or out of consideration for others. In addition, the names of some of the individuals have been changed for reasons of privacy.

Introduction

✦

2007

In 1968, when I was seventeen, I joined the Army to get away from the troubles at home and volunteered to go to Vietnam.

In 1970, at nineteen, I returned home, a drug addict and alcoholic with undiagnosed Post Traumatic Stress Disorder. I spent almost three decades trying unsuccessfully to get clean and sober. My journey led me to a stay in a mental hospital, to so many detoxes and drug treatment centers that I lost count of the number, to numerous jail confinements, three terms in prison, and three suicide attempts. I lost my home, my family, my job, my self-respect and any hope I'd ever had that I could live a normal life. I owned nothing, not even the shredded, filthy clothes I wore.

In 1998, at the age of forty-seven, I was living in a cardboard refrigerator box in downtown Tampa, Florida, when a miracle happened.

Four years later, in 2002, I had professional career as a Zone Manager at Bay Pines Veteran's Affairs Hospital in St. Petersburg, Florida, where I was supervising almost fifty employees; I owned my own home and car, and had more friends than I'd ever had in my life.

My story is not about being strong enough to pull myself out of terrible poverty and addiction, and fighting to succeed against all odds. Mine is a story of barely holding on to a ragged thread of hope in the face of decades of defeat and humiliation; of finally learning that surrender and acceptance worked for me when running away or fighting back didn't; of learning how to take thoughtful, deliberate action to change my life and become the man I always wanted to be.

Going through recovery has been the hardest work I've ever done and rewarding beyond anything I could ever have imagined. I've done my best to honestly explain my motivations and feelings when I was using drugs and alcohol, as well as my thoughts and fears as I went through the process of recovery. My hope is that sharing them will help others understand addictive behaviors and the healing process. For me, facing my fears and understanding my emotions have been the most important keys to changing my life.

I have a mental image of myself at nine or ten, watching sailors walk through our dirty, gray neighborhood in Portsmouth, Virginia, talking and laughing over the noise of the shipyard. I'd think to myself that nobody could really be as happy as they seemed to be. At last I have those things I dreamed of when I was a boy. Today my life is filled with love, trust, and self-respect. I've learned to deal with problems instead of allowing them to control me.

I wanted to write this book to encourage others to recognize that ordinary people can succeed in the face of seemingly insurmountable odds. If I was able change my life, you can change yours.

A Box Called Home

✦

1998

I figured it was ants crawling on my arms and face in the sweltering heat of August 1998, but I didn't want to look. Opening my eyes would make everything worse. I rolled over and groaned. My head ached. Close by, eighteen-wheel semis roared down Channelside Drive in the shadow of Tampa's skyscrapers—they weren't helping. Ants. It had to be those fucking Florida ants.

Shit. I brushed my hand across my cheek and felt them swarm all over me. I tried to sit up inside the sagging cardboard refrigerator box that had been my home for the past two weeks. I inhaled the sweet smell of stale alcohol, and with my eyes still closed swatted the ants away. No matter how many layers of cardboard I put between me and the ground, those goddamned bugs always found me.

Finally I opened my eyes and felt the familiar sharp pain as the light hit them. Squinting, I brushed myself off, then hunted for the spot where the ants were coming in. I didn't often find a box big enough for my six-and-a-half foot frame, but it helped that at the age of forty-seven I only weighed about a hundred and twenty pounds. This was the best refrigerator box I'd ever had but I knew it would only last till the next hard rain. After two thunderstorms, one side was about to cave in. I looked through the window I had cut in it and saw a white man dressed as a security guard headed my way. *Oh, shit,* I thought.

"Hey," he yelled. "Who the fuck you think you are? You get your black ass outta here!" He came over and kicked the box hard.

I scrambled out, holding my hands up to shield my face from the sun. I said, "Hey, man! I ain't hurtin' nothing. I was just resting." But what I thought was, *Fuck you! You think you're better than me. If I was white you wouldn't have said nothing.*

"You get off this property," he yelled. "And don't let me catch you here again, you fuckin' no good bum."

"Yeah, yeah. You have a nice day, too," I said.

I dragged my refrigerator box behind a clump of bushes, hoping nobody would steal it before I got back. Then I reached for my raggedy backpack that held only a hairbrush and an ink pen, stumbled around the corner and sat down hard on the curb, holding my aching head in my hands. The thought of having to live through one more day this way was more than I could stand. I'd existed in deep, dark despair for years. I'd been alone my entire life. Nobody cared whether I was alive or dead. Why did I even bother to live? I heard myself say out loud, "I just can't do this no more. I got to change my life."

In the back of my mind, I'd always thought I could call my parents for help as a last resort. But my mom had died two months earlier and I was too ashamed to call my dad. I was sure he wouldn't even talk to me. I couldn't go back to live with my half-sister Ivy, either. She was supposed to be holding my share of the money we had inherited from our mom's death insurance, but Ivy had her own drug problems so I really wasn't surprised that she'd disappeared.

Exhausted and desperate from always having to sleep with one eye open, never having enough money, enough food, enough drugs or alcohol, the only thing I could think to do was to return one more time to the Department of Veterans Affairs (V.A.) Hospital. But I remember thinking, *What's the point? That shit don't work for me.*

I had a few coins in my pocket that I'd saved from my last day labor job so I could buy a beer for breakfast. Instead, I forced myself to go to a nearby pay-phone and use the money to call my V.A. rep.

The receptionist who answered said my social worker wasn't there but a college intern was covering for her, so I asked if I could talk to her. I told her my story and she said she'd have to look through my file and then see if she could find a bed in one of the detox centers.

"That's great." I said. "I'm not sure what name they have me under. My real name is Eugene Hairston, but I've always gone by Billy. So it could be either one of those."

"Thanks, I'll look under both," she said. "Now I want you to know I'm new here." She sounded excited, like she was determined to do a good job. "I haven't done this before, so it may take a while, but I'll do my very best to locate something for you."

"That's fine, I'll stay right here on the phone while you look," I said.

"No, no. Let me call you back. I don't know how long I'll be."

"But," I said, now desperate to hold onto the connection, "but … I won't be able to call you again. I only got a quarter."

"Don't you leave that phone," she said. "I'll call you back even if I can't find anything. Don't you go away."

"No, no. I'll be right here," I said, and gave her the number. It sounded like maybe I was her first case, and I hoped she had lots of good help. I remember thinking that in a way, maybe it was good my social worker wasn't there. I'd fucked up so many times with her she probably would have blown me off.

As I waited for what seemed like forever, a man came up and stood behind me. I knew he could tell I wasn't talking to anybody, so I looked at the ground like I didn't see him and hoped he'd go away. After a few minutes he said, "Hey, Mack, you gonna use that phone or you just gonna stand there?" I looked up and gave him a weak smile, but he just glared at me.

"I'm waiting for a really important call, man. Sorry. It'll be just a few minutes," I said, and turned away from him. He finally walked off. When the intern called back twenty minutes later she'd found me a bed in a detox, several miles north on Nebraska Avenue. "Go right now," she said. "Right this minute."

An overwhelming sense of relief flooded through me. "Thank you, thank you," I said. Immediately, I picked up my backpack and started walking toward Nebraska Avenue. I looked back toward my refrigerator box, thinking I should hide it better, but then thought, *The hell with it.*

I'd gone a few blocks when a familiar thought sneaked into the back of my mind. *I ought to earn some money from day labor before I go in. I only got a quarter.*

I shook my head and forced myself to keep walking. *No, if I don't go to treatment now, I never will.*

I tromped along for another block thinking, *I really need a little money. I don't even have cigarettes. Maybe I could find a half-day's work today and start treatment tomorrow.*

Then on the next block, *No, I might lose my spot. When I get money I just buy drugs.*

My mind was stuck again on the treacherous and unbearably familiar treadmill. Should I or shouldn't I?

I got to the treatment center about 10 a.m. and gave the receptionist my name. "We have your referral but you'll have to come back later," she said. "We don't take new patients till 5 p.m." I looked around the room for a place to sit and she said, "You'll have to come back. Sorry. We need those chairs for visitors." I stepped back from the counter and looked down at my feet. *A seven-hour wait in this heat,* I thought. I walked outside into the sweltering August day and stared at their sign, "Community Alcohol Treatment Center."

I had nowhere to go so I headed for a sunny bus stop bench across the street. I sat down and watched the traffic whizzing by. I hadn't eaten since the dry bologna sandwich they'd given me at day labor the day before; my mouth was sour and dry, my stomach cramped and my hands were shaking. I thought about what I usually did every morning—buy some crackers and a beer at a convenience store and if I was lucky, steal some cigarettes. The thought of popping open a can of cold beer made my mouth water. That first cool one always deadened the needles that jangled every nerve in my body and calmed the shakes. But I only had a quarter.

I leaned forward on the bench and looked at the sidewalk. Ants, like the ones that always found me, marched along by my foot. One of them struggled with what looked like a crust of bread ten times bigger than he was, and I thought to myself, *That's like me. Weighed down. Barely making it. But at least he's got a piece of bread.*

The old mental treadmill reappeared. *Maybe I shouldn't go to treatment now. I could go to day labor instead. I've got nothing to do all day but sit here. Maybe I could get a day job and be back here by five.*

Then I'd think, *No, I won't come back. When I get any money ...*
But detoxes, they expect you to come in drunk anyway.
But I might not get back.
On the other hand ...
Then again ...

After an hour or so, a man carrying a drink in a small brown paper bag came and sat down beside me. I could tell by the colors on the can that it was a tall Budweiser. I heard the metallic "pop" as he opened it and at just that moment the bus appeared. When he walked toward it, the driver signaled that he couldn't bring the beer with him. He came back and put the beer down on the bench beside me. He had not even taken a sip. He got on the bus.

My head throbbed in the steaming heat and my stomach ached. That beer was so cold the paper bag was wet. I looked at the treatment center and I looked at the beer. I looked back at the treatment center and again at the beer.

I reached out my trembling hand. *What could one beer hurt?*

Choices

✦

1968–69

I was seventeen, living with my mom and eight-year-old half-sister Ivy, in Portsmouth, Virginia. My school grades were failing, I argued constantly with my mom and Ivy, and my friends were fed up with my drinking. Something had to change. I came home late one Saturday morning after staying out all night and flopped down on the worn brown sofa in the living room of our small apartment. The stale smell of alcohol and cigarettes hung in the air as my mom cleared catsup-covered dishes and dirty glasses from the table where people had been drinking the night before. The income from her "bootlegging" business supplemented what she earned cleaning houses; it brought in enough money to keep us fed but not much more.

"Where the hell you been?" she asked, looking over at me. "You know you got a curfew."

"I'm thinking about joining up with the Army," I said.

She glanced at me sideways and kept stacking dishes. "Is that so? Hummph. Well, your father made a career out of the service." She wiped the table with a dishrag. "Might be a good chance for you to see the world."

"And maybe I could send you some money to help with Ivy," I said, feeling generous because she wasn't yelling at me.

"No, now, Billy Junior, you just take care of yourself. I got along this far without no help." She stacked the glasses, one inside the other and put them on a pile of plates. "If you can send me something then do, but don't you worry none about it."

"You'll have to sign for me," I said.

She looked at me again, wiping the table more slowly. "You know, I think getting out of this town would be good for you. The Army would teach you some discipline."

"You'll sign for me then?"

She smiled like she'd be glad to have me far, far away and out of her life. "'Course I will. When you be leaving?"

The next day my Aunt Lena called. When I heard her voice on the phone a calm feeling came over me. She was the only person in the world I felt had ever really loved me. "Your mama told me you thinking about joining up with the Army," she said.

"That's right."

"Now, Billy Junior, I ain't telling you what to do, but I want you to think hard about it. We don't want you getting hurt or killed or nothing. You need to think about it and pray to ask for God's direction. Don't want nothing bad happening to my Billy Junior."

"I got to change something, Aunt Lena," I said. "Mom is always yelling at me, I never do anything right; everything's just in too big a mess."

"You need to think about finishing high school first," she said. "You need your education. You ain't going nowhere without an education."

"I know, I know," I said. "I can go to school when I get out. Even go to college on the GI bill, they said. This is really what I want to do."

She sighed. "Well, all right then. I pray that God'll watch over you like he did when you was little and got so sick," she said. "He'll keep you safe. My God is a powerful God."

"Thanks, Aunt Lena."

"You know your Aunt Lena loves you, now."

"I know," I said. "And I love you, too."

I thought about telling my father that I was planning to sign up, but since I hadn't seen him in a year or so I decided against it. He'd been in the Navy and I was sure he'd just put me down for joining the Army. I'd never once in my life done anything that pleased him. *Nah,* I thought. *No need to tell him.*

I told my girlfriend, Bett, what I was planning and she thought joining the Army was a great idea, a good reason to throw a party. I knew her dad would be glad to see me go. He was a preacher, very strict about everything she did, right down to the clothes she wore. For some reason, he thought I was a bad influence on her.

I told the rest of my friends that I was planning to enlist and the next weekend one of the girls threw a party for me. Bett said she'd meet me there and I rode over on the bus with my friends Clint, Leroy, Buck, and Vernon. Our parties were always loud and long, and as usual we all drank too much and smoked too much weed.

We stayed till about two in the morning and because the buses weren't running we had to call a taxi to get home. Since none of us had any money, Buck came up with a plan.

"All right," he said, "Here's what we're gonna do. I'll call the cab. We'll get four of us in the back and Clint, you sit up front. When we get to the projects, we all get out of the cab and make like we're looking through our pockets for the fare. Then when everybody's out, we all run in different directions. Ain't no way he can chase us all."

"Sweet," Clint said, and we all gave each other five.

"Hey, man," said Leroy, "I can't get caught doing nothing wrong. My ass is already on the line. If I get caught …"

"No way," I said. "You can run faster than some fat ass cab driver."

Leroy frowned and said, "All right. But I'm gonna sit next to the door, not in the middle."

Everything went fine till we got to the projects. As Buck was getting out of one side of the taxi, Leroy jumped out the other side and ran down the street like the devil was after him. The driver pulled out a gun and aimed it at Clint, "Move and I'll blow your fucking head off," he shouted.

I climbed out and ran with the rest of them, but when I looked back Clint was still in the cab. I felt bad for him but I kept on running. He called me from the police station after I got home and said, "Hey, Billy, that fuckin' cab driver called the cops. Sure as hell he'd have shot me if I tried to fight him."

"Shit, man. That sucks."

"Listen here. They're saying there were three cab robberies tonight and they're trying to pin 'em on me."

"No way."

"You gotta come down here and tell 'em I was at that party and it ain't me."

My stomach knotted up. "But, say, man. If they find out I was in on the cab deal they'll arrest me too."

"Hey, Billy. I could go to prison for this shit. And I didn't do none of it."

"I know, man. I know. I'm coming. I'm not gonna let you go out like that."

Before it was all over, the girl who'd given the party brought her mom down to the police station and they told the officers that Clint had been at the party all night. In the end, we were both charged with theft of the cab fare. For some reason they didn't care about the guys who'd been with us and we didn't bring it up.

The idea of going to court scared me, but I'd heard that the first time might not be too bad. I didn't like having to stand in front of the judge but I'd dressed real nice and tried to look responsible. He read the charges and said, "How do you plead?"

"Guilty," we both said.

"Guilty," he said. "All right. I see the original charge was armed robbery but there was insufficient evidence. I see neither of you have a record. Are you working? Going to school?"

Clint said, "Thinking maybe we'd go into the Army. We been talking to a recruiter."

"Well, that's a good idea," the judge said, leaning back in his chair. "That sounds like a fine solution. You heard of the 'Buddy-Buddy' plan?"

Clint and I looked at each other and back at the judge. "No sir," we both said.

"If you enlist with a friend, you can stay together from Basic Training to Advanced Infantry Training. That sounds like a good option to me," he said, looking from one of us to the other. "I'm going to be generous with you. I'm going to give you the option of serving two years in the penitentiary or three years in Uncle Sam's Army. What do you say?"

I looked at Clint and we both turned back to the judge. "We'll take the Army," I said.

The next day we were on a bus to Richmond, and the evening after that we were on a train to Fort Benning, Georgia.

There were about a thousand military recruits with us on the train that night, so it was no big surprise that the club cars ran out of liquor. Most of us looked like we were between seventeen and twenty, ranging from big country boys to skinny city slickers. There were geeks wearing glasses and even a few in suits. It was clear that most were excited to be off on a big adventure and many of us were drinking to celebrate our entry into manhood. Clint played dice with the other guys, but I just got blind drunk and passed out on one of the seats.

"Hey, Billy! Wake up." I heard Clint whispering as he yanked on my shoulder. "Look what we got here!"

I pulled away. "Leave me alone, man. I'm sleeping."

"Come on, Fool. All these guys are passed out. We can get paid! Go into their pockets and they'll never know a thing."

I opened my eyes and squinted at him. "What time is it?"

"Shhh," he said, looking at his watch. "Almost four. We got to work fast!"

I sat up and looked around the darkened car at the men passed out in the seats, snoring loudly. A lot of them were even lying in the aisle. The stink of sweaty bodies, cigarettes, drink and vomit turned my stomach. I wiped my mouth and shook my head to get it clear. "Phew!"

"This is sweet, man," Clint whispered. "Look." He went over to one of the guys lying on the floor, pulled all the cash out of his wallet, then replaced the empty wallet. Then he got a money clip from a guy slouched over in his seat, stuck the bills in his pocket, and put the clip on the floor, like it had dropped out. I dragged myself to my feet and fumbled my way up the aisle. It was my first and only train robbery.

When we reached Fort Benning an hour later, a drill sergeant got on the train yelling at the top of his lungs, kicking the men who were still asleep. "Move it! Move it! Fall out and line up! Now!!" We all stumbled out of the passenger car to the sounds of the sergeant marching up and down, barking, "Everybody off your ass and on your feet," and "Move it, move it, move it!" and "Grab your gear, you motherfuckers." Men were tripping over each other as we all ran to the military transports.

"Hey, Sergeant," I heard one of them yell, "My money's gone."

"Well now, that ain't my problem, is it?" the sergeant answered.

"Me too," another man called. "My money's go …"

"Shut up, you sissies," the sergeant shouted. "I ain't got time to listen to your shit. You're in the Army now. Line the fuck up."

"But, sir," another one said.

"Sir?" the drill sergeant said. "I ain't no sir! I work for a living!"

"But …"

"You hear me? Move it, move it, move it!" Kicking and pushing us, he said, "You hear what I told them morons? You get the fuck in formation before I take your wallets and shove 'em up your asses! Now!"

Some of the men were angry, but we all did as we were told.

"Move it, move it, move it!" the sergeant shouted. "Get in the back of the truck, now! Move it!"

When we got to the base we were assigned to a platoon of a hundred men, most with hangovers, red-eyed and rumpled with stunned looks on their faces. We stood at attention with our backs to four two-story barracks, while the sergeant barked orders at us. "I want you assholes to take your gear into the barracks behind you, go to the first or second floor," he said, pointing to the building behind us. "Pick out a bed, stow your gear, and be back down here in three minutes flat. You punks got that? Three minutes flat!"

He paced in front of us. "Listen up now, shitheads. Before you go in there, right inside that door is the center deck, right between them white lines. No one steps on my center deck, at no time! That's mine! I polished that goddamned deck and I don't want none of you dirtbags putting even one little scratch on it, you understand?

"Yes, sir!"

He shouted, "I told you scum not to call me sir!! You call me Drill Sergeant!!"

"Yes, Drill Sergeant!!"

"If anybody puts one little tiny mark on that deck, the whole fucking company is gonna pay, you hear me?"

"Yes, Drill Sergeant," we called out.

"Can't hear you, assholes."

"Yes, Drill Sergeant," we yelled louder.

"Ready!" he shouted.

When he held up his watch and blew his whistle, we grabbed our gear and raced into the building. Beds were lined up along each wall with a locker at the foot of each one. There was a white stripe on the floor the length of the building, which was even with the foot of the beds. The center deck he was talking about was the area between those two lines, which you would have expected to be the walkway most often used. We all raced in, trying to avoid his deck. "You got two minutes!" the sarge yelled. Then, "One minute, you maggots. Get the fuck down here."

When we were back in formation, the sergeant walked up the steps of the barracks, then leaned forward, his hands on his knees. "Somebody walked on my center deck," he shouted. "Thought I told you candy asses not to put any scratches on my center aisle. Didn't I?"

"Yes, Drill Sergeant," we yelled.

"I can't hear you!"

"Yes, Drill Sergeant!" Nothing we said to a drill sergeant was ever loud enough.

"Well, some of you shitheads walked on that floor anyway, didn't you?"

Nobody said a word.

Louder. "Didn't you?"

Someone shouted, "Yes sir!"

"WHAT!!" The Drill Sergeant ran over to the guy and got in his face, nose-to-nose, and yelled, "Do you see bars on my collar? I work for a living. I'm not your fucking mother, father, sister, girlfriend, or wife. You can and you WILL call me Drill Sergeant!"

"Yes, Drill Sergeant," the poor guy said.

"I can't hear you," he bellowed.

"Yes, Drill Sergeant," we all shouted.

"Now drop soldier, and do push-ups till I get tired."

The sarge repeatedly slapped his baton hard against his hand, stuck out his chest, and strutted back and forth in front of us. With an evil smile he yelled, "You're the dumbest bunch of fuck-wads ever to come to this base. There's marks all over that goddamned deck in there … after I told you not to enter that center aisle. So ladies, here's what we're going to do. The whole fucking lot of you are gonna crawl on your bellies, down across this gravel," he said, pointing at the parking area. "You're gonna crawl 'til I get tired. You hear me?"

"Yes, Drill Sergeant!"

"I can't hear that weak shit!"

"Yes, Drill Sergeant!" we yelled.

"Then we'll see if this'll help you girls remember to follow orders!"

"Yes, Drill Sergeant." A few of the men started getting down on their hands and knees.

"Down!" he shouted. "Now! Right this fucking minute!" The rest of us got down with the guy doing push ups and started dragging ourselves over the gravel, bitching about who'd run on the floor and what we'd do to them later if we could find out.

We repeated that drill two more times before we could go inside without leaving a mark on the center deck. Each time we failed, we crawled for what seemed like hours. Five guys passed out and three went to the dispensary that night. Only two of the three returned.

Late that night Clint and I went in one of the bathroom stalls and counted the money we'd lifted that morning. We were fat! Instead of having ten dollars in my pocket to start basic training, I had five hundred.

◆   ◆   ◆

We woke up each day to the sound of garbage can lids being slammed together and the sergeant yelling, "Move it, move it, move it, you punks! Get your fucking asses outta here. Only thing comes to a sleeper is a dream."

Within five minutes we were dressed and in formation out front, standing at attention. The sergeant yelled constantly, "Move it, you got two minutes you maggots, you motherfuckers. Get your candy asses out here. One minute! Move it, move it, you dip-stick SOBs."

For the first week we ran five miles in formation before breakfast and after that every other day the miles were increased by one. The first few days I was bent over double by the time we got back, barely able to catch my breath. We all spent a lot of time bitching about how sore we were.

After the run we'd clean up and get back in formation to go to breakfast. We were always busy, all day every day, at target practice, physical training, cleaning our rifles, or policing the area. Every time one of us fell short, we all suffered.

There was one huge white guy we called "Soul Pig" who was from the back woods of Alabama. He was always the last one to drag in from the morning run, the guy who didn't have his comb and soap in exactly the right place in his footlocker during inspection, the one who forgot to shine the back of his shoes. Every time somebody screwed up, and it was usually Soul Pig, the sarge made us all drag ourselves through the gravel for an hour or crawl under the barracks and "raise the roof" which meant to yell as loud as we could. No matter how loud we bellowed, he called us pussies and sissies and told us we were weak and to shout louder.

In the beginning we were pissed off when the sarge called us all those names, but because we were all in it together it seemed to get easier. The fact that Soul Pig was the one getting us into all the trouble didn't get easier though. Some of the guys hated him for it.

One day Soul Pig accidentally called his rifle a gun and the Drill Sergeant went crazy. He grabbed the rifle and shouted in Soul Pig's face, "This is a rifle! This is for shooting!" Then he grabbed his crotch. "This is my gun! This is for fun! Now, everybody drop and give me fifty."

For the first week the men threatened to beat the shit out of Soul Pig, but after that we began to see that he was really trying to do better but just couldn't. Gradually, we realized that if we wanted to stop crawling through gravel and "raising the roof," we were going to have to help him. During the morning run one guy would carry Soul Pig's rifle, another one his backpack, and two ran along beside him to keep him in line. We'd inspect his rifle and help him stow his gear properly. We even took him drinking with us.

Around the middle of the second week about five hundred of us were standing in formation before going to breakfast when the sergeant asked, "How many of you morons don't have high school diplomas?"

Over half of us raised our hands, including Clint and me.

"All of you with your hands up," he said, "right after chow, you report to Building D. You're gonna get your big chance to become high school fucking graduates."

When we got to the building, there were rows of tables and chairs set up; a test booklet had been placed in front of each chair. The test was multiple-choice with questions about American history, geometry and reading comprehension. I did the best I could, but it had been a long time since I'd actually tried to pass a test. I was sure I failed.

After supper the next night, I was walking up the stairs in the barracks and heard Soul Pig shouting over the other men, "You asshole! What you taking out my locker? You stealing from me?" When I got to the door there must have been forty men sitting on bunks or standing around cheering and calling out to Soul Pig and Clint.

"I didn't take nothing out your locker," Clint said. "I just opened the wrong one, that's all."

"Yeah?" Soul Pig said. "Well, what you got in your pocket there if you didn't take nothing?"

"I ain't got nothing, you retard. You calling me a liar?"

"Hey, come on now," I said, walking into the room, "Cut it out."

"You're goddamned right you're a liar," Soul Pig shouted, "I seen what you was doing." Soul Pig held his fist up in Clint's face, never a good idea, and Clint went after him.

"Hey," I said, heading toward them. "Stop it. What the hell you doing?"

Clint hit Soul Pig hard in the face, and the big man staggered back but didn't fall. He came back at Clint like a train.

"Come on," I said to the men standing around watching. "Help me stop this."

"Oh, no, not none of me," one said. "I want to keep on living, myself."

"No way, man. They're too big," another one said.

By this time Soul Pig and Clint were trading blows pretty good. I could see that I was the only one who was going to try and stop the fight, but it was just because I knew Clint wouldn't hurt me. I jumped between them. "All right, now. That's enough. You two break it up."

They were stepping apart just as the sergeant walked in. "Atten-Hut! What's going on here, boys? What we got here?"

Soul Pig said, "Nothing, Drill Sergeant."

Sarge just looked at him.

Soul Pig stared back, his lip bleeding. Then the sergeant looked at Clint. "You, again!" he said, narrowing his eyes. "You just got yourself two weeks on K.P. And you," he said, glaring at Soul Pig, "you just got two weeks cleaning latrines. See if you can figure out the difference between the sinks and the urinals. And you can both start now!" the sarge yelled. "Right this fucking minute!" Clint and Soul Pig looked at each other with hatred, but neither one made eye contact with Sarge as they walked out of the room.

As soon as they left, the sarge turned to the rest of us. "Ladies," he said. "I have an announcement to make. I just got the scores back from your GED tests, and only one of you morons passed. We got us one genius out of two hundred and seventy of you degenerates. What a bunch of dip-sticks."

We knew better than to ask who it was.

"We have only one man in this here barracks who could have gotten out of high school. No wonder you're such a bunch of hopeless pricks. All but one." He stopped speaking again and looked around the room. Then he said, "Hairston, front and center."

I couldn't believe it! I knew it had to be a mistake but I started over to him.

"And because of that," he said to the rest of the men, "and the fact that Hairston here was the only one with balls enough to stop that fight, I'm promoting him to Squad Leader." He shook my hand. "You'll get Temporary Sergeant's Stripes for this."

I remember thinking I wasn't as dumb as my mom had always said I was. It was the first time I'd done something I considered important, all on my own. There had been high school basketball, but I was just part of the team.

Then I thought about how pissed all the guys were going to be who hadn't passed the test. I knew they'd kid me and maybe even fight me over it and told myself I'd need to watch my step. But I was happy to write my mom about it. Maybe she'd be proud of me.

So this was the beginning of my military career, me and Clint on the Buddy-Buddy plan. We continued to raise havoc, running crooked gambling games with loaded dice, and hustling guys by playing Dirty Hearts. Clint stayed in trouble, and as the Squad Leader, I tried to cover for him.

◆   ◆   ◆

Henry Marlow, one of the guys we played cards with, was our Platoon Leader. He'd been discharged from the service months before and was living in Atlanta. By some mistake, he'd been called back up and had to work on the base during the day for the two months it took to straighten out the paperwork, but he didn't have to live on the base. Henry just wanted to get back out of the Army and was always ready to go out drinking with us on weekends.

"Hey, Bro," he said one morning. "My girlfriend's coming to pick me up tonight. You and Clint want to cruise Atlanta with us?"

I was always ready to go. "That's cool. I'm down," I said. "But I ain't got a lot of cash."

"You know somebody in the bar always gets a soldier his first drink," Henry said. "And somebody else will buy you the next one. Then we'll go to another bar and start all over again."

We went lots of times, usually driving into town with Henry, but since he didn't have to return to the base till morning we'd catch a bus or find somebody to give us a ride back. Eventually the night came when we couldn't hitch a ride to the base and we had to go home with Henry. In fact that happened several times, but we got him to drive us back early and we were already there before the garbage can lids started clanging.

Exactly one week before we finished Basic Training, we spent the night at Henry's, and the next morning we were all still too drunk to drive to the base. That time Clint and I were caught AWOL and I lost my Temporary Sergeant's Stripes. *What the hell*, I told myself. *I'll be outta here next week.*

Everybody looked forward to graduation and we all drank to celebrate. We talked about how tough we were, and how we'd kick some ass when the time came. The night before the ceremony, we found out that despite our help, Soul Pig didn't make it—he was going to have to repeat Basic. That was a big disappointment because we'd done our best to help him pass.

Clint and I were both assigned to Fort Ord in Monterey, California for Advanced Infantry Training (AIT), where Clint ended up going into cryptography, which required a high security clearance, go figure, and since I'd done well on office skills, I was sent to be a Company Clerk. Because we were in different units, we didn't get together much after that, except on weekends.

I worked as a Mail Clerk for six months and was offered a permanent position with the top sergeant there, but in the end I decided I wanted more excitement and transferred to Fort Campbell in Kentucky. There I hung out with a unit of battle-weary men who had just returned from Vietnam. Every night in the bar I listened to their wild, exciting stories and decided that was for me. Within a few weeks, I volunteered to go to Vietnam.

The Smell of Diesel Fuel

✦

1970

On Feb 1, 1970, I arrived at Tan Son Nhut Air Force Base in Vietnam. I was assigned to "A" Company and went through the 1st Cavalry Training Academy where we were taught, among other things: rappelling, how to safely board and disembark from helicopters, and how to find trip wires. We completed jungle training and learned about the customs of the Vietnamese people. We also learned the gooks were experts at crawling through the miles of concertina wire the Army laid out. They'd use two little metal rods to pry the coils apart just wide enough to crawl through. They were small people, so it was easier for them than it was for many of us. To combat that problem, we were taught to set flares under the wire that would go off if someone tried to get through.

A month later I was onboard a C-130 Cargo/Passenger plane with about two hundred other men, coming in for a landing in Ben Hoa. Looking out the window, all I could see was the lush green canopy of the jungle. Then, suddenly, we were over what looked like an empty patch of dusty gray asphalt. When we landed, the rush of heat felt like it had come from a blast furnace.

We were all hurried onto waiting buses, and as we pulled away from the plane we heard sharp cracking sounds, then a thunderous, "Boom! … Boom! Boom!"

My stomach lurched and I bent forward in the seat as far as I could. The driver stepped on the gas and yelled, "Get down!!"

One of the guys in the rear shouted, "Oh, my God! They just blew up our fucking plane!" As the driver slowed, we all looked out the back. Black smoke was billowing out from the C-130 we had just left.

"Welcome to Vietnam," the bus driver shouted over his shoulder, and hit the gas again.

When the buses pulled up to the orientation site, the overwhelming stench of burning diesel fuel and body waste hit us like a wall. Smoke ballooned from barrels that had been pulled from underneath the latrines and set on fire. The smell reminded me of a soap factory near my house that burned its refuse every week and I expected the odor would soon be gone. But it turned out that the smell was there twenty-four/seven. While I got used to it, like everybody else, I was always aware of it.

There must have been close to a thousand of us new recruits that day and they crowded us all into a big building. The Captain who was in charge called out over the loudspeaker, "Everybody who's been trained for 11 Bravo and 13 Charlie—that is trained for combat—raise your hands." About three hundred hands went up. Then he asked, "How many had training in other MOS?" (Military Occupation Specialties) The rest of us raised our hands and I could tell by the look on his face that this was not what he was expecting. He turned his back to us and talked to the officers standing behind him, then faced us again and said, "All right men. Listen up. I'm dividing you into two groups." He lifted his arm and made an imaginary line dividing one quarter of the men on the right from the rest of us. "You'll all have temporary assignments, those on the right will go to administration support and everybody on the left to combat support, that's the 11 Bravo, 13 Charlie MOS supports." Unfortunately, I was on his left. I ended up temporarily assigned to Flight Operations Support.

At the Supply Hooch we got our M-16s and ammunition. As I held the rifle, I was reminded of the toy rifle and the jungle outfit my Uncle James had given me when I was a kid. Now I had the real thing and I hoped I could become the man I'd pretended to be back then.

"Now remember, you morons," the Captain said, holding up his M-16, "This ain't a gun. This here's a rifle. Keep it clean. It'll save your life. It's your best friend."

I stood there, holding that rifle and listening to far-away explosions and the whomp, whomp of helicopters as they came and went. I felt ten feet tall. *I'm the man,* I thought. Then almost instantly, panic hit me. I thought, *This is for real. People die here. I could die here.*

When we finished the Cavalry Training Academy a week later, I was assigned to the First Air Cavalry, Air Mobile, Aviation Battalion. When I learned I was going to be part of a helicopter aviation unit I thought it was really cool. I'd heard some of the guys back at Fort Campbell bragging about flying big Chinook 47s, Huey CH 13s and Mosquito Observers—how they'd outsmarted the bad guys and saved each other's lives. I daydreamed about doing the same things, being respected and doing something important.

But I also remembered another guy at Fort Campbell. He'd just returned to the states and he sure as hell didn't feel like a hero. One night he got really drunk, curled up on the floor of the bar and cried like a baby. He talked about being right next to his friends when they were blown to bits, and their blood and brains were splattered all over him. He'd been terrified he was going to die. Those memories would sneak into the back of my mind and I'd think to myself, *Don't be such a coward.* My stomach would clench into knots and I thought I'd puke, but I tried to focus on the hero part.

Later, as we flew in to our assigned Fire Base Landing Zone (LZ), I stared down at what looked like a big ugly brown-gray scab on the earth. It was a nasty little clearing that had been burned out of the green jungle with fiery napalm, like we'd seen in pictures while we were in training. The sun glinted off the steel roofs of the hooches and the big rolls of concertina wire that surrounded it. A heavy blanket of dread fell over me and I thought, *This is nothing but a fucking dump. Why in God's name did I ever come over here?*

◆   ◆   ◆

Our hooches were windowless buildings made of sandbags with corrugated steel roofs. Mats hanging from the ceiling served as walls, which gave us some privacy, but the air was stifling. Mosquitoes buzzed everywhere and bit us right through our clothes. I was constantly slapping my neck and face, and any other exposed skin.

I met Ace and Slim, both new recruits like me, when we were all assigned to the same hooch. Ace, a short, dark-skinned muscular brother, came up and said, "Hey, man, gimme some Dap." He stuck his hand out and I reached to shake it. "No, man. Dap. Gimme some Dap."

"What's that?" I asked.

"Here, let me show you."

He put out his hand and showed me the basic handshake. Two men slap the palms of their right hands together three times, and then curl their fingers inward, making a loose handshake. Then, they pull and push three times, raise their hands over their heads, and slap palms together again. The whole thing comes together in one fluid motion. Ace said, "What's up, Brother?" and I answered back, "Brother be good."

"You can add your own stuff to it," he said. "but that's Dap. It was started by the black brothers over here, and now everybody in Vietnam does it."

To me, giving Dap came to express love, brotherhood and support. It was a universal acknowledgement that we'd been in a place that separated us from the rest of society. It meant much, much more than a simple handshake. It was a single sign of unity.

After we stowed our gear the three of us went to the mess hall. I grabbed a tray and stood in line but the food looked runny and lumpy, like white slop. "What is this?" I asked the Vietnamese man who was spooning it out.

He nodded at me and smiled, showing teeth all black from chewing betel nuts, and said, "That food. Good America food."

"But what is it?" I asked again.

He looked at the guy next to him and said something in Vietnamese and then laughed. "Food. Good food." Then he waved his hand at me to move along.

Ace curled his lip. "I ain't eating this shit," he said. "You can't even tell what the fuck it is." He picked up his tray, slammed it down on one of the tables and left, but Slim and I stayed in line.

I looked behind the Vietnamese cooks and could see that our meal had been prepared in huge pots. Fly strips hung all over the mess tent, with trapped flies still buzzing away, struggling to escape. The cooks wore black pajamas with the pant legs rolled up to their knees, and their calves and feet were covered with mud and dirt. A couple of them were squatting on the floor, chopping some vegetables on small wooden blocks. The floor was covered with spilled food and drinks and looked like it hadn't been mopped in weeks. The cooks spoke to each other in sharp voices, talking loudly, showing those black teeth. I had the feeling they'd be likely to spit in the food and I'd heard some of the guys say they might feed us rat poison.

When I finally tasted my meal, I decided it was runny macaroni and cheese, and tasteless, limp, gray-colored green beans. Within a week, most of the guys I knew bought freeze-dried lerps or C-Rations or even canned goods at the Post Exchange (PX) and cooked them on hotplates.

When the sun went down, it was absolutely pitch black; I couldn't see further than a few feet ahead. It took me straight back to the times when I was a kid and my mom locked me in a closet for a few hours as punishment. Back then, my eyes adjusted enough to the light that I could see a little, but in Vietnam the darkness was unrelenting. Since the enemy was all around us, at night we could have no lights on within the camp boundaries that could be seen from the outside; even jeeps were driven without headlights. But huge bright spotlights faced out from the camp, flooding the jungle that surrounded us with light. They were placed on the berm that surrounded the LZ; that way we could see the enemy but they couldn't see us. Sunset came early because tall trees surrounded us, blocking out most of the sky. Dusk became the worst time for me because I knew blackness would soon follow. I hated those pitch-black nights.

We slept under mosquito netting and the droning of insects put me to sleep. I bought four small battery fans at the PX that I kept going all the time, two at the head and two at the foot of my bed. It didn't take me long to learn how to get dressed under that netting.

◆   ◆   ◆

I hung out mostly with Ace and Slim. Ace was from Texas, a hot-headed mechanic who was always ready to beat somebody up. He never backed down from a fight and sometimes even went looking for one. He'd hold his fist up and say, "When I get back home and some white honkie wants to shake my hand, he can just shake my fist. No open-handshake for me."

Slim was light-skinned and tall and thin like me and told us he'd joined up to get away from Philly. He was easygoing, always telling jokes and writing letters to his girlfriend.

Ace is the one who gave me the nickname I still carry. Because I'm so tall, he started calling me "Tree" or "Treetop."

The first week we were there Slim, Ace and I, along with two other guys, were assigned to help build an Enlisted Men's Club, a canteen where everybody would be able to buy sodas and five percent beer, play a little pool and shoot some darts. Samuels, the white supply sergeant who supervised the construction, explained that first day, "I got stuck with this fucking job, and we're gonna get it done as fast as we can. I ain't putting up with any shit from you morons."

"They gonna sell cold beer?" Slim asked.

Samuels sneered at him. "We're gonna build a stage right over here where we can have some of the locals perform and show movies," he said. He walked back and forth as he talked, explaining.

"Cool," I said.

He ignored me. It was clear he didn't like dealing with black men, and the fact that none of us knew how to build anything didn't make it any easier. He showed us how he wanted the work done and we got started. Samuels got more and more hostile as the days passed, yelling and calling us stupid fuck-wads. We couldn't do anything right. Every night Slim and I had to talk Ace out of killing the guy. It took us about two weeks to complete the club, and they were stocking it with beer and cold drinks before we'd finished. While we were cleaning up the unused building supplies, I asked Samuels, "When's this place gonna open? I'm ready to shoot some pool."

"You ain't gonna be doing that, Hairston," he said. "It's off limits to you."

"Off limits? What you mean, off limits?"

"I mean that's just the way it is here, motherfucker. No niggers allowed. You'll have to get used to it. You and your kind can sit in the bleachers outside and watch the shows or buy beer at the window, but you ain't coming in."

"You can't do that," I said, anger rising inside me. Then, louder, "You can't fucking do that." Ace and Slim and the two other guys started walking over.

"Just watch me, fella," Samuels said, and shot us a bird as he walked away. We all stood there, stunned, not wanting to believe what we'd just heard. But rage quickly took over.

"What the fuck is this shit," Ace said, throwing a hammer against the side of the club. "We built the fucking place."

"We're goddamned good enough to die for our country but can't go inside and have a beer?" Slim said. "What the fuck is this?"

All of us came back to our hooch and sat around for two hours trying to figure out what we could do. "Man, it don't do no good to fight them," Slim said. "Just get yourself killed, you or somebody else. Just do your time and go home in one piece."

"No way!" Ace said, so mad that he couldn't stop pacing. "Them goddamned assholes ain't getting away with this."

One of the others yelled out, "Right! Them cocksucker honkies—we'll kill 'em all."

"Now, wait just a fuckin' minute," I said. "Remember, we ain't in the world, here. We're in Vietnam. Everybody here's got a gun and we're way outnumbered."

"Listen, man," Ace said. "We ain't got no choice. We ain't taking this shit." He hit a fist into his other hand.

"Right," I said. "We ain't taking it, but it don't make no sense to fight back with guns. They'll just kill us all and hide it."

"Yeah, you're right, bro," Slim said.

"They'll wipe us off the map and cover it up," I said. "You heard the stories. Then they'll tell our families we got killed in an ambush. I ain't going out like that."

"All right," Ace said, standing in the doorway. "Then we'll rope off our section and won't let them honkies get anywhere near us."

"So, asshole, how you gonna keep them out?" one of the other men said.

Ace held his hands up like he was aiming his rifle at us. "If they come in here we'll shoot their goddamned stinking motherfucking balls off. Eh, eh, eh, eh," he said, spraying us with imaginary bullets.

"Naw, man," I said, lighting up a cigarette. "We gotta fight smart. There's more of them than there is of us, so we gotta think. Use our fuckin' heads. Every day blacks and whites go out together on sorties and we all watch each other's backs. You know that's the truth."

"Yeah, bro. That's the truth," Slim said.

"Now you know most of the pilots and door gunners are white and the mechanics and supply staff are black, but they work together."

"That's right, Brother Tree."

"And it takes everybody to bring our men back alive," Slim said. We talked on and on, and when we couldn't agree on what to do, we did nothing.

A few days later everybody on the LZ was encouraged to come to the first movie they were showing at the club. Slim and Ace and I brought some drinks and something to eat, and sat in the bleachers with about twenty other black guys. We were in the back rows, off to one side, while about a hundred whites were sitting in front of the screen. The night started out with a stripper who did her thing with a smoking cigar, something I'd never seen before, while everybody shouted and whistled. Then they started the movie.

It opened with two big, fat white men standing in the main road of a small southern town accusing a gray-headed black man of stealing a sack of flour from the grocery store. They shoved him back and forth between them, saying, "Boy, ain't you got no respect? We don't tolerate no thieves around here, nigger."

The whites in the audience cheered them on, "Get that uppity son of a bitch! Hoo Boy!! Get that fucking nigger!!"

Then the white sheriff came in and slapped the old man around while the other two held him, and the audience yelled even louder, "Come on, give it to that motherfucker." It was one of the most racist movies I've ever seen. All of us black men sat there, once again not believing what we were seeing. I kept thinking that maybe it was one of those movies where the bad guys start it off and the good guys come in and put them to shame. But that wasn't happening.

When the old man's little grandson came to help him they grabbed him too, and shoved him around. The sheriff spit in the boy's face and the kid just stood there as the spittle ran down his chin.

Most of the white soldiers were yelling and cheering when somebody pitched a beer can at the screen. All of us black guys joined in, throwing food, drinks, bottles, anything we could find. Then, almost as if it had been planned, we all stood up at the same time and went after the men who were shouting. Immediately, it was a riot, a free-for-all.

The fight probably didn't last long, but it felt like it did. The Captain started shouting through a bullhorn, "Disperse Immediately! You men are ordered to disperse immediately! Return to your hooches! On the double!" It took a while for everybody to calm down and in the end, the black men, who, they said, had "started" the fight, were restricted to their hooches after 8 p.m. every night.

Ignoring the curfew the following evening, about ten men came to our hooch, where again we argued about what we were going to do. When things started dying down, somebody mentioned the Inspector General, the I.G. and it rang a bell in my head. I said, "Hey Brothers, I've got an idea. I learned a few things when I was a Company Clerk back in the world. I think I know what we need to do."

"Let's hear it, Bro. We gotta do something," Ace said, standing with his arms across his chest.

"It wouldn't have worked before because it was just our word against Samuels'. But everybody at the movie saw this. We got to go to the I.G. Tell him what's happening."

Ace rolled his eyes.

"How do we do that?" Slim asked.

"I'll write him a letter. Don't nobody have to know who wrote it, but I'll get it off tomorrow. And I'll tell him about everything: the canteen restrictions, what the food is like in the mess tent, the movies and the curfews just for us."

"But if that don't work we're gonna kill them sons of bitches," Ace said, pounding his fist into his other hand.

"Okay, Ace," I said. "But let's just try this first."

I wrote the letter and sent it off the next day. I never got an answer, but within two weeks there was a surprise inspection by the I.G. team and all hell broke loose. In addition to our complaint, other serious problems were uncovered. As a result, the Captain and the First Sergeant left the base and the Mess Sergeant was demoted. Samuels, the Supply Sergeant who wouldn't let us in the Enlisted Men's Club, was found to have falsified records and didn't get the promotion he was up for. He was enraged and we all loved it. The restrictions on the club were lifted but as far as I know, none of us black men ever went back over there. Sometimes when Ace was in a mood to stir up some trouble, he'd say, "Hey, let's go throw a few darts. Show them honkies who's who." But even he knew better than to do that.

Although the name of the person who wrote to the I.G. was supposed to be kept secret, everyone seemed to know who did it, and Samuels didn't try to hide the way he felt about me.

◆   ◆   ◆

During the daytime, Vietnamese people were all over our base. Our "hooch maids" were women or boys who were allowed into the LZ every morning to clean for about two dollars a day; floors were swept, clothes were folded, dishes were washed, and beds were made. They cleared away any litter that was outside and even did a little landscaping; to cut the grass several of the hooch maids squatted down in a row, each with a pair of scissors, and moved across the yard together, snipping away.

Some of the women were whores, but only a couple of those girls would be let in each day. Most of the prostitutes hung out at a place called the Psychedelic Shack, where men called papasans or boys called boysans pimped for them.

There, soldiers could buy hamburgers and beer as well as sex. It was about a mile away on the Thai side of the LZ and was run by a mamasan named Maya, who was about thirty years old. She was short and dark with a plain face, not what you'd call attractive but she had three pretty girlsans and two boysans working for her. One day I was over there having a beer with some of my buddies when Slim said, "Hey, Tree. Why don't you give Maya a poke?"

"Aw, naw, man," I said, lighting up a joint.

"Come on, Tree. Twenty bucks says you won't do it."

"No way, man," I said, shaking my head. "She's not right for me."

"I'll give you fifty," Slim said, reaching for his wallet.

"Make it a hundred and you're on," I told them.

They looked at each other and Ace said, "We're down." They each put fifty dollars on the table. "Go for it, man."

I went up to Maya and pointed to her and to me and made a motion with my hands. She shook her head and said, "No do. No do. Pick pretty girlsan."

"I want pretty Mamasan," I said, and the girls with her started giggling. Maya got an angry look on her face, but she took my hand and led me to the back room.

When I returned to the table and collected my money, the guys gave me a hard time. Then food and drinks started turning up. "I didn't order this," I said to the boysan. "No, no. We no order."

"You no pay, you no pay," the boysan said, with a big grin.

Slim reached over and hit me on the arm. "Hey, man. Guess you rocked her boat!"

I smiled. When we were leaving Maya came over and pulled me to the side. She said, "You no pay. You no do any girlsan. You do only me. I do only you." She didn't ask me, she told me.

Two nights later I heard a noise in my hooch and grabbed my M-16. It turned out to be Maya and two of her girls who had sneaked onto the base. "What the fuck you doing?" I asked her. "How'd you get in here? I could' a killed you."

"Shhh," she said. "I come see you. My girls here for your friends."

"Okay," I said as she crawled under my mosquito netting. "But be quiet. I could get in a lot of trouble."

◆   ◆   ◆

New recruits at our LZ were mostly eighteen to twenty years old, usually without high school diplomas, and many had been in trouble with the law at home. This type was considered good for the military because they were more gung ho and were also considered expendable; many were lost during their first month in country. Losing friends in combat was really hard on the men, and many who had been there a while wouldn't make friends with the new guys; they waited to see who lived through the first month before getting attached to anybody.

To go to sleep and to stay awake, we took drugs, which were easy to get. We bought heroin and cocaine from some of the papasans when we were on "hops" to other areas. I tried opium once and even used what they called purple heroin—which we later learned was rat poison. I sprinkled a little on some weed before I smoked it, but I didn't get much of a reaction.

Alcohol was everywhere but the ability to get it depended on your rank. A Buck Sergeant or higher could buy liquor but those below that rank could get only five percent beer and sodas. Since the temperature was usually one hundred and five to one hundred and ten degrees and drinking beer just made us sweat more, most of us preferred reefer, which was cheap and available. It gave us energy and made us feel mellow, which helped take away some of the fear.

What Have I Done?

✦

1970

My first assignment was Crew Chief. I was trained on the job by Ernie Patterson, a crew chief on a huge Chinook 47 helicopter. Patterson made it clear that I'd be responsible for everything that goes on in the belly of the helicopter, from deciding who would get in to loading and securing equipment.

I was stationed at the gunnery port in back of the co-pilot, behind an M-60 that was fastened to a rod embedded in the floor. I couldn't shoot without orders to do so, and as it turned out, the only thing I shot at was water buffalo, which we killed to limit the gook's food supply.

On the second day of training we took off with the regular crew of five men, and went to pick up some equipment at a remote site. After we landed, a man in a brown Korean Army uniform ran up to Patterson and, in broken English, asked for a hop back to the base; he and his buddy had two prisoners who, they said, wanted to defect. Patterson told me they often gave hops to the Koreans, and he okayed them to get on board after we loaded up.

When we finished securing the equipment, Patterson nodded to the Korean. The man then called over to a nearby Quonset hut and another Korean soldier walked out with the two gooks. The North Vietnamese prisoners were dressed in black pajamas, their hands tied behind their backs. The Koreans shouted at their captives, shoved and kicked them while the men cowered and turned away; one of them was young, maybe a teenager, and the other looked old enough to be his father.

I knew the Koreans had been in a terrible battle the week before and a lot of their men were killed. They were out for revenge and everyone on the base was talking about how losing so many of their men had made them crazy. They'd slaughter any gooks they could get their hands on, so I was surprised they were even taking prisoners.

When the crew was ready for take-off, the Koreans boarded with the Vietnamese men and shoved them into the fold-down seats that ran along the sides of the belly of the helicopter. The pilot climbed into the cockpit, looked back toward us and said, "This is going to be a rough ride, guys."

I sat at my gun port as we lifted off and looked for movement below. When I heard our passengers yelling wildly over the whomp, whomp, whomp of the copter blades, I turned to look at them. I had no idea what they were saying, but the Koreans took turns slapping the older man across the face till he was a bloody mess. I turned back to the M-60. When I heard scuffling and a short scream, I looked back again and watched as the old guy was dragged to the open bay in the back, a machete held to his battered face. It looked as if he had been cut. He tried to twist away but the Korean kicked him, then stabbed him over and over and shoved him out into the air. The Korean kept stabbing the air with his knife even after the prisoner had disappeared from sight.

I was stunned. *That didn't just happen,* I thought. *That didn't happen.*

I called over to Ernie, "Hey, man," but he just waved a hand without even looking directly at me, as if to say don't get involved. I wanted to do something but it was too late. Prickles of dread pierced my skin; I was full of adrenaline but frozen to the spot. I couldn't believe it, but at the same time I knew what I had seen. I turned back to my M-60 and stared out over the treetops determined not to look toward the back again. When we landed twenty minutes later, the kid was still there. He must have given them the information they wanted.

As we walked away from the helicopter, Patterson came over and said, "What happened today don't go no further, you got it?"

"But …" I said.

"You heard me, Treetop. You want to forget it, trust me. It's not fair, it's war."

When Patterson walked off ahead of me, the pilot came up and put his hand on my shoulder. "Chill, Tree. No big deal. They do worse to us. Put it out of your mind."

As he followed Patterson, I stared at their backs. We had just witnessed an atrocity of war. We might not have actually participated but we allowed it to happen. We could have stopped it. That scene will be forever embedded in my memory.

I witnessed a number of atrocities in Vietnam and heard about many more. In fact, what the rest of the world called atrocities, to us were just everyday acts of war. Most of us were just kids ourselves and acted out of fear, rage, and immaturity. We did things we'd never have done at home. It was in Vietnam that I learned the true meaning of the old saying, "You can't really judge a man till you've walked a mile in his shoes."

◆   ◆   ◆

Besides our regular assignments, everybody took four-hour shifts at guard duty. We were trucked out to huts that had been built on the berm, an elevated area surrounding the perimeter of the camp. Each hut was about four feet high, covered by a corrugated tin roof and had sandbags piled on top. There was an M-60 in each hut and we brought our own weapons along; all in all, it wasn't too bad when it wasn't raining.

Our job was to stop anyone from crawling through the concertina wire or getting into the camp. We reported any sounds or sightings to the Sergeant of the Guards, who was in radio contact with us every ten or fifteen minutes. Once in a while he'd send us a signal or code to kick back to him, to verify that all was well.

Helicopters and patrols went out twenty-four/seven, napalm was dropped night and day, and sometimes animals set off flares trying to get through the concertina wire. In the dark they were all terrifying. Some nights the explosions were almost constant. I never got used to that.

At first, when things were slow, we sometimes threw stones through the wire to set off the flares planted there, just to relieve the boredom. After they made us crawl through the barbed wire to replace the flares, we stopped doing that.

When we called the sergeant to say we'd had a sighting or heard some unusual movement out in the bush, they flooded the area with lights and dispatched a helicopter. We also did that once in a while when it was too quiet—created a little excitement to keep everyone from falling asleep. We avoided sleep at all costs because it was very possible that someone would be trying to sneak in. But most of the down time was spent smoking reefer and talking about home and family.

"When I get back, I'm gonna start my own business," Slim said. "Auto repair shop. I got a way with cars."

"You talked to your little lady about that?" I asked.

"Shit, man. She'll go along with anything I want to do. That gal's crazy about me. Just can't get enough."

"Yeah," I said. "I know. My Bett's just the same. Mmmm. Some sweet thing."

"Just wait till I get back," Slim said. "I got plans. Big plans."

"I'm gonna give my mom some money to get a house," I said. "She's worked hard all her life. It's the least I can do. Or maybe I'll get her a new car. The one she has must be fifteen years old."

"She'll go for that," Slim said.

"Yeah, man. That's what I'm gonna do."

As time went on and we knew each other better, we actually came to trust each other. That was new to me. Until then, the only person I'd ever really trusted was my Aunt Lena.

We had a lot of down time on guard duty and that's where we often shared the things closest to us, the pain when our girlfriends left us, our anger at the fathers who had abandoned us, and our rage at the cops who were always ready to grab a black man. We shared our disappointments, the hard times we had growing up poor and black, our fears of dying in a foreign land, and frustration about how we were fighting in Vietnam when we should be at home, active in the Civil Rights Movement.

But when I was just sitting around the hooch talking, I usually said what I thought the others wanted to hear because I wanted to be accepted in the group. I laughed at things that weren't funny, like hearing that a place back home had been robbed or that the police had killed somebody. I felt lost, so for the most part I just did my best to fit in. In the back of my mind I still wondered if Vietnam might be the place where I could make my mark, maybe even go home a hero. But the reality was extremely harsh and painful. The gruesome fact, that men died every single day, was constantly with me. Tomorrow it could be one of us. Tomorrow it could be me.

When napalm was dropped it sprayed burning phosphorus, killing everything it touched and leaving a scorched black ruin and the stink of death. Many days, having to continuously inhale the horrible smell of fuel oil and burning human waste was overpowering. It polluted my entire body.

We were there, of course, to kill as many North Vietnamese as we could and life was very cheap. We watched as our "killer teams" attacked the gooks using an observer helicopter and a gunship. They'd send a small bubble observer copter over an area they thought might be inhabited by the enemy, to entice them to shoot and give away their position. When they fell for it, a big Cobra helicopter followed the smaller one and demolished them. As we sat on the berm and observed the process, we'd eat our meals and talk with each other as if nothing was going on; as if people weren't nearby. It was business as usual. Killing the enemy was supposed to be cause for celebration, and I acted like I was glad. But late into those dark, black nights I thought about the people we'd killed that way.

◆   ◆   ◆

Mail call was the high point of every day for most of the soldiers and getting even one letter was enough to raise my spirits for a week. When I didn't get anything for a while I'd pull out the old letters and read them again. I heard from Bett every few weeks, but mostly her letters were filled with stories of how awful it was at home. Her mother had been sick with diabetes and that scared her, she never had enough money, and school was too hard. If that wasn't enough, there were race riots and our people were constantly being mistreated. A few of our friends were hurt in riots; one was even killed. What I needed to hear was good news. Here I was, fighting for my country on the other side of the world, and I wasn't treated any better than they were at home. Other black men got letters like mine, which made many of them want to strike back at the whites around us. But still, any letter was better than no letter.

I was surprised to get a birthday card from my mom, and for Christmas she sent me a package with a rum cake, a box of turtle candy, peppermint balls, chewing gum, and four pairs of socks. I couldn't believe she had sent so much and knew that Aunt Lena must have had something to do with it, probably even bought some of the stuff. My mom had often told me that I was a mistake and should never been born and I'd long ago given up any hope that she would ever love me. But however it happened, for a while I felt like I was one of the guys with a family who missed him.

◆   ◆   ◆

A week or so after I'd been trained for Crew Chief I was transferred to a new assignment, Dispatcher, reporting to the Flight Operations Commander, Jimmy Acton. The move was a surprise, and it later occurred to me that it might be the result of what I'd seen. They probably knew I'd already written the I.G. once. Whatever the reason for the transfer, I was glad to take it.

When I started on-the-job training, I was immediately overwhelmed. The stress was unlike anything I'd ever imagined. Every single day men's lives literally depended on information I passed on to them. Me. An eighteen-year-old kid.

My code name was "Polybird" because I passed information back and forth between the pilots and Acton. This included troop movements, confirmations, locations of supply drops, hot and cold zones, and pick-up and drop-off zones. Acton plotted each warrant officer pilot's flight plan, but the tactics changed constantly. The pilots had to keep him informed of their whereabouts and activities. They relayed their coordinates when the gooks shot at them and had to get his permission before they could shoot back.

For the eight months I was a dispatcher, I sat in a well-lit hooch in front of a bank of crackling radios and transmitters. Every morning briefings were held where new code names were assigned to each helicopter. This was to keep the gooks from using our transmissions against us. When a lot of sorties were planned, a second dispatcher was on duty.

Acton stood right behind me, feeding me information and putting colored pins in a map to keep the locations straight: red for gook sightings, blue for villages, yellow for bodies, etc. As a dispatcher I worked two to five sorties at any given time, and some individual sorties had six or more helicopters assigned. Pilots requested data constantly and my giving them the right coordinates and positions could make the difference between life and death.

It was a couple of months after I started the job that a second dispatcher, Rudy Vasquez (Vaz), was called in because of the heavy action expected that day. We had been working since 5 a.m. without a break; it had been five hours of hell. The action was non-stop and one of our birds had gone down. For most of that time we'd been listening over the radio to the voices of terrified men screaming above the sound of the helicopters, "Got incoming. Shit, where did they come from? Did you see 'em? Did you see 'em? Oh my God, I'm hit! Oh, God!"

I felt helpless—shaking, sweating, sick to my stomach—desperate to do something to help them. Men were dying. I was hearing their last words. And all I could do was listen.

It was at least a hundred degrees in that hooch by 10 a.m. I wasn't surprised when Vaz started flipping out. He stood up and ripped off his earphones, then slammed them down on the desk. "I can't do this, man. I can't do this no more."

"Hey, Vaz," I said, leaning back in my chair and doing my best to sound calm. "Chill out, man."

"This is fucked," he said, getting up and pacing. "We need more radio hams. I can't do this."

Acton stopped Vaz and held him by the shoulders. "We're all we got," he said. "Get a grip, now. Tighten up. You ain't goin' nowhere."

A voice came over my radio and above the roar of the helicopter I heard, "Charlie Hector 386 to Polybird. Coordinates Lima Alpha 926 124. Got three little Indians down."

"Roger," I said. "Three little Indians. Lima Alpha 926 124. Need a nurse call?"

"Roger, Polybird. On the double." I heard shots and explosions over the roar of the helicopter and, as always, my stomach lurched. Sweat ran into my eyes and I wiped it away. The pilot yelled back, "Fuck! Those guys are in bad fucking shape. Shit!"

"Copy that, 386. We're getting a med response." I wrote down the coords and handed them to Acton who picked up a receiver to call. "Got a clearing where they can set down?" I asked.

Acton, behind me, yelled into his receiver, "Got three down. Coords Lima Alpha 926 104."

I turned to Acton. "The coords are 124, not 104!"

"Got it." Acton shouted into the phone, "Correction. Coords Lima Alpha 926 124. That's 124, not 104."

"386 to Polybird. Don't look too fuckin' good," the pilot said. "Charlie's everywhere."

Acton leaned over my shoulder and wrote down some numbers. "Here's a clearing," he said. "Medicvac's on the way."

"386. Tell 'em to get the wounded to Lima Alpha 926 113. We'll have a medicvac there in ten minutes."

"Roger that, Polybird."

Just then Vaz kicked the trashcan hard. Garbage went everywhere.

"Hey, man," I said. "What the hell!" Vaz was shaking all over, sweat dripped from him and he looked like he was about to collapse. "Come on, man," I said. "We'll get through the day."

Acton's face turned red and he frowned. He stormed over to Vaz. "What the fuck is your problem! What the fuck you doing! I got two down and a lost ship. You get your shit together or I'll get it together for you."

Vaz wiped his face with both hands. Taking a deep breath, he turned back to his radio and sat down.

Acton grabbed a sheet from the Teletype machine. "We got to deal with one world at a time," he said over his shoulder.

When Vaz got his earphones back on I leaned back to Acton and whispered, "Hey, man, Vaz got a Dear John yesterday. Didn't get no sleep last night. Probably thinks he'd be better off dead."

Acton shook his head.

"Sometimes I do too," I said under my breath.

"Drop one of them BT pills and mellow out," Acton called over to Vaz. "We got no time for breaks. We got birds out there."

Vaz looked at me with red, teary eyes. His hands were still shaking. "Come on," I said, handing him some pills from my pocket. "Two more hours. You can do it."

The radio brought me back to the job. "Polybird, this is 143. We dropped a blue flare on that jeep we lost, and we're up, up and away. That line went snap, crackle, and pop, man. Got some ants down on the ground who'd be able to pick her up?"

"Roger that, 143. I'll check and get back to you."

"Polybird to 2nd of the 12th, you got a ear on? Need you to check out the blue smoke cloud. Got a jeep down. Baby in a hot spot."

"176 to Polybird. Come in." Then I heard, Boom! … Boom, Boom!! I jumped, every nerve in my body tight enough to rip apart.

"This is Polybird, 176. You guys okay?"

"176. Just circled around to pick up six little Indians but we can't see any-body. Don't look good. There's a lot going on down there. You heard anything?"

"I'll check, 176. Hold on. Got one ahead of you."

"Recon 2nd of the 12th to Polybird. We were en route to the sheep." He paused and screamed, "Cover that right flank! Where the hell is Dave?" Then he spoke to me again, "Fuck, it's hot out here. Got two down." His voice broke and he shouted, "I gotta get the fuck outta here. I said close that flank!" Then, "Need a medicvac. We can get to Lima Omega 106 296."

"Polybird to 2nd of the 12th. Gotcha." I wrote down the coords and handed them to Acton. "Hold on. Medicvac's on the way." Then I turned to Acton, "Two down. Lima Omega 106 296."

"Polybird to 143. Forget the jeep. Only ants in the area got two down. Let it go."

"This is 143. Roger that, Polybird."

Acton shouted, "Polybird, tell 176 dee dee mal! Get outta there! Charlie's out and about! Just north is a hot zone! Head to Lima Omega 106 137."

"Copy that. Polybird to Uno Siete Seis. Dee dee mal! Get the fuck outta there. It's hot. Shake ass to Lima Omega 106 137."

"Polybird, this is 176." Men screamed frantically in the background, some-body crying, "Oh my God, my leg! I'm dying, I'm dying."

"Polybird to 176. I'm here."

"176 to Polybird. Confirm pick up seven little Indians. Two down …"

"This is Polybird. Roger that."

"Polybird, this is 243. We went to drop off food supplies at Lima Alpha 355 842. There ain't nothing there, man. No camp or nothing. Just a clearing. What you want me to do?"

"Hold on," I said, and turned toward Acton. "243 says there's no signal and no smoke at the site where we told him to drop supplies. I got him down at Lima Alpha 355 842."

"Drop it," Acton said. "That's right. Tell 'em to drop it."

"But," I said, "there's no ..."

"Drop the fucking thing!" he yelled.

I turned back to the radio. "Sarge says drop it."

"Polybird, this is 243. Don't look right to me. Something's fucked up, man. But if you say so."

When our replacements showed up around noon, Vaz and I went back to my hooch and smoked some weed. The joints we rolled were the size of cigars, much bigger than the ones we smoked back in the world, so it didn't take us long to mellow out. Ace and Slim came in later with some sodas and we smoked reefer and played cards till midnight.

◆   ◆   ◆

After several months I knew without a doubt that very often the information I gave pilots wasn't what had been on the morning flight plans. It didn't take a genius to see that something wasn't right. For example, Acton would have me tell a pilot that a jeep, scheduled to be dropped off at another LZ, should go to a remote clearing somewhere out in the jungle instead. Or I'd give the pilot a manifest ordering three hundred pounds of flour to be delivered to a site, then an hour after it was dropped off I'd get a call from the site saying they only got a hundred pounds. I talked to my buddies about how some of our field units were missing supply shipments, which didn't make me any friends when it got back to the officers. It wasn't until I was back home in Portsmouth that I learned of the widespread black market operating there, that equipment was regularly sold to the Viet Cong and the Russian friendlies. Then it all made sense.

But what was worse, Acton had me tell pilots to fly through areas we knew were hot, without telling them about the danger. This happened repeatedly, even though I was always asking him, "Sarge, you sure about those coords?"

He always answered the same way. "Polybird, you just read what I give you. You're here to follow orders. Don't ask no questions and you'll be fine." But I knew men were getting injured, maybe even killed after following some of the directions I gave them, and I felt responsible.

Almost every evening somebody came to my hooch and questioned me about the coords or something I'd given out that day. I was lying on my bunk, reading a mystery one night when Derek, one of the crew chiefs, walked into my hooch and said, "Hey, man, I want to talk to you. That was some fucked up shit that happened today. What the hell are they doing up there in operations? That mission was whacked."

I sat up and turned to face him. "Hey, man. All I know is what they tell me. That's all I can pass along."

"Know those coords you gave us? We took incoming but you didn't give us no word it was hot."

"It wasn't given to me. I didn't know it, man. I'm just a Polybird. I repeat what they give me, but I don't set the sorties or the routes. I don't know any more than you do."

"But you're changing coordinates, and we don't know what the fuck is there when we go in. This is some foul shit. That crap can get us DOA'd or make us fire on our own men," he said, shaking his fist. "If I find out I'm risking my life for some bullshit or some money, I'm gonna fuck somebody up. And my word is my bond."

"Hey man, I always double-check when it don't sound right but Acton tells me what to say. What can I do? If I knew something better to tell you, I'd do it." I held up my hands and leaned back. "You guys know I'm straight."

"We need some motherfuckin' answers," he said.

"You're right," I said. "Why don't you report it to the I.G.?"

"Yeah. This company's track record ain't that hot. I ain't going down like no punk, for no bullshit. Something better happen quick before we decide to change things."

"I know, man. It sucks."

"Maybe I will report it to the I.G. Think it'll do any good?"

"Can't hurt."

He turned to leave. "Thanks, Treetop," he said. "Look out for us."

I felt bad but I knew that as the middleman, I didn't have the answers they needed. It didn't take me long to get very distrustful of my superiors.

After Derek left I went over to the Psychedelic Shack for a cool one, and before I even sat down Maya called me into the back room. She took my hand and pulled me over to the cot to sit beside her. She smiled and looked straight into my eyes. "I have boysan," she said, pointing to her stomach.

"Huh? What?" I said, moving away so I could look directly at her. "You what? You mean you're knocked up?"

She nodded her head several times, then smiled and pointed her finger, first at me and then at herself. "Yes, Tree. I have little Treetop."

"Huh? What? How do you know?" I asked, standing up. "Did you go to a doctor?"

She stared at me like I was the dumbest person in the world. She took a deep breath. "You mansan," she said, pointing at me and nodding her head. Then she pointed to herself, "Me girlsan. Me know."

"Oh, well, um." I'd never even thought of this. I had so much else going on it just never seemed a possibility. Panic spread over me. I couldn't handle one more problem. "I got to go," I said. "I got to get back. We can talk about this later."

She didn't move, just sat on the cot and looked at me. Her smile faded.

I didn't know it then, but that was the last time I'd ever see her.

◆   ◆   ◆

Early the next morning I was covering for the mail clerk, who was on R&R. I got a jeep and drove to the helicopter pad where the mail came in. I grabbed our mailbag and was headed back when I saw three choppers headed my way. As they crossed over the perimeter they started receiving incoming mortar rounds, "Boom! … Boom, Boom!" In a panic I hit the gas, thinking *Shit!! This could really be it! I could die!*

The rockets missed the copters but one exploded nearby. My jeep flipped over on its side and I was thrown clear. I'm not sure how long I lay there but men ran over and dragged me off to the side of the landing pad. I was numb, felt nothing. I had no idea how badly I was hurt.

They put me on a stretcher and hauled me to the closest MASH Unit for treatment. I'd caught shrapnel in my left knee and my right lower calf, nothing life threatening but it was painful. Still stunned, I lay there while the doc cleaned and bandaged both legs and wrapped the right one in a soft cast. After giving me a pair of crutches, they discharged me back to my unit with orders for light duty and bed rest. They called my company for somebody to pick me up and I sat down out front. As I waited, my mind kept wandering back to the incident but I pushed it away, trying to just stay with whatever was right in front of me. *I'm alive*, I thought. *That's what counts.*

A Cloud of Bees

✦

1970

I sat out in front of the MASH tent for over two hours, waiting for someone from my company to pick me up. The nurse had called three times, but still there was no response. Finally, it seemed to me that the fastest way to get back to my command post was to walk. So, around noon, in the sweltering heat, I started out on the six-mile hike. On crutches. I figured I'd be able to get a ride from a passing jeep but there was no traffic at all. The land was bare from all the defoliants, so there was no shade on the dusty road. I slogged along, covered in sweat that made my hold on the crutches slippery. My right leg ached. Occasionally I got dizzy enough that I had to sit down and rest, but I didn't stay long because the heat was even worse when I wasn't moving.

I was about halfway back and very sorry I'd ever decided to try to walk it, when I saw a jeep from my company headed toward my post. "Thank you God," I said out loud. "Thank you God." I stopped and turned, waved my crutch and yelled, "Hey! Here! Hey, stop!" The jeep didn't slow down. I waved harder and yelled louder. The driver turned his head the other way as he sped by. It was Samuels. That motherfucking son of a bitch Samuels, the Supply Sergeant who ran the canteen, the guy who missed his promotion because of the I.G.'s surprise visit.

I stood there in the swirling dust, boiling with rage. "You SOB! You motherfucking SOB!" I shouted. Tears streamed down my face and my whole body began shaking with the huge sobs. *Stop it*, I told myself. *You're a soldier now. Stop it, you coward.* But I couldn't. I screamed out to the empty road, "AAGGGH-HHH!!" and sat in the dirt.

Finally, with tears and sweat streaming down my face, I got up and hobbled on. By the time I finally limped up to the company office to report my return, I was so exhausted I could hardly stay upright. Three men were standing around the entrance, smoking. The only one I knew was Samuels, who was leaning against the wall, blowing smoke out through his nose, smiling at me. A surge of rage exploded inside me. I hobbled up to where he stood as fast as I could. I lunged for him. "Goddamn you," I yelled, swinging my crutch at him. "You no-good son of a bitch!"

He held his hands up and backed away, easily deflecting the blows. But something inside me snapped. I couldn't stop swinging at him.

The C.O.'s clerks came out and grabbed my crutches. I went after Samuels with my fists. They grabbed my arms. Wild with rage and pain, I fought back.

Finally, they dragged me inside and shoved me into a chair. I gasped for air while everybody stood around, watching the show.

"Okay, Buddy, take it easy. Calm down," someone said.

"Why didn't you pick me up, you fucker?" I shouted at Samuels.

"What you talking about? Pick you up?"

"You saw me on the road." I looked from Samuels to the other faces around me. "I just walked here from the MASH Unit because nobody from this fucking place would come and get me," I shouted at them. "They called three fucking times! Look at me! I've been wounded! I took shrapnel in my leg this morning and that son of a bitch drove right past me on the road."

"I never saw you," Samuels said, with a smirk on his face. "You're imagining things."

From the chair, I lunged at him again but the others grabbed my arms and threw me back into the seat. "You motherfucker," I yelled. "I'm reporting you to the I.G.! We'll get this straight!"

By this time the Company Commander came in and all faces turned to him. "I been listening to all this. Hairston, you're confined to your quarters till further notice. Bailey," he said to his clerk, "take this man back to his hooch."

I was getting shafted again. "Do you know what he did?" I yelled.

"Just shut up!" he said. "I don't need to hear nothing out of you now. You have attacked a non-commissioned officer. Go back to your hooch."

Bailey walked over and said, "Pick up your crutches and walk, Buddy." He escorted me to my hooch in silence, then left. I rearranged my now bloody bandages and an hour later I was lying on my bunk with all four fans going, drinking a soda, replaying the morning's events in my mind. I looked up when I heard someone coming.

Bailey appeared in the doorway. "Captain says you've got orders to ship out, so pack up your gear."

"I don't know nothing about no orders. Where are they?"

"Captain says he don't have them yet. They'll be shipped to your new station."

"No way, man," I said, shaking my head. "I'm not going nowhere till I get written orders. What kind of sucker you take me for?"

"I'm telling you to pack your gear, Tree, and I don't want no trouble."

"Listen, I know I have a right to see the paperwork, and without that I'm not doing a fucking thing. You can tell him that."

"You're pushing it, Tree. They're out to get you, man," he said as he turned and walked away.

I got up and checked some of the nearby hooches but everybody was gone. Panic rose in my chest. I thought, *What in God's name am I going to do?*

Finally Slim walked in and pointed to my bandages. "Hey, Bro," he said. "I heard what happened. Are you okay?"

When I finished telling him what had gone on, his face looked deadly serious. He said, "Let me tell you something, Tree. About nine or ten months ago, there was this medic who was a brother. He was this cool dude everybody called Doc, and he was the first one to complain about the way we been treated out here." Slim looked me right in the eye. "One day just out of the blue, Doc said he'd been transferred to another base, but they didn't give him no orders either. They made him pack up his gear and he left that same day. Doc didn't think it sounded right, but hell, he didn't know what else to do."

I didn't say a word but my stomach clenched into a knot.

Anyways, he always wrote his mom every week, and every week she'd send a box of cookies and fudge that he shared with us. Not long after he went off, I wrote to his mom, asking where he'd been transferred. She wrote back saying she got papers listing him as MIA."

The knot in my stomach cinched tighter. "So what you think happened?"

"Well, add two and two. He pissed off the honchos and he's flying in a chopper. Maybe he fell out when it's five hundred feet up. Maybe he got sent out on a sortie and they forgot to bring him back. Maybe he just accidentally caught some friendly fire. Don't matter now. We all know he's dead, but he's still classified MIA."

"Shit!"

"Looks to me like you're in line to end up just like him. Listen, man, everybody's over at the Psychedelic Shack getting with a unit that's on stand down. I'll go get 'em. Be right back."

After he left, I sat on the bed and tried not to panic. Everything was going to hell. Slim had been gone about twenty minutes when Bailey returned, this time with a forty-five.

"Get up and pack, Tree. You're leaving."

"I ain't packing nothin'."

"Either you pack or I'll do it for you. Orders from the C.O."

"I don't care who they're from. I ain't packing shit and get the fuck off my ass, Bailey. I don't want to hurt you, but I will."

About that time we heard the chugging roar of a Duster, a vehicle like a small tank. I turned and to my great surprise and relief, I saw Ace leading the charge with Slim and about fifteen other guys from the Psychedelic Shack all waving their weapons and yelling. As it pulled to a stop, the men ran up with their firearms.

"We're with you, Brother Treetop. You ain't goin' nowhere," one of them yelled.

"Fuck this bullshit. They ain't getting' away with this!" Ace shouted.

"Hey, Brother Tree, you stayin' right here. All for one and one for all. We'll die together."

My sense of relief was overwhelming. I choked back tears. I'd been saved from an execution. The men ran in close and surrounded me, passing Dap to each other. Then I saw a face that didn't belong there. I looked more closely and was amazed to see that the driver was a guy named Java that I'd grown up with in the projects in Portsmouth. He ran up and hugged me, then gave me Dap, and then another hug.

Java said, "We'll get you back home, Brother Billy. I mean, Brother Treetop. What the hell you doing here? I didn't know you was the one they was talkin' about!"

"Hey, man," I said, giving him more Dap.

"We're just here on a two-week stand down," he said. "Looks like you got your ass into some shit, huh?"

Out of the corner of my eye I saw Bailey leave. A few minutes later a bullhorn blared out. "Put down your weapons," the voice said. "You men are ordered to disperse immediately."

Everything got quiet and I looked up to see Samuels standing beside Bailey, about ten yards away.

"Put down your weapons, I said. Now! Hairston, you report to the C.O.'s office. On the double."

Nobody moved.

The men started yelling back at him. "You assholes crazy. Tree's not goin' nowhere."

"Bring it on."

"Tree ain't leavin' here. You'll have to kill us all first."

I had never in my life gotten that kind of support. Those guys were ready to die to protect me.

"Wait!" I yelled at the men around me, and waved my crutch. "Wait a minute. Let me talk to 'em." They kept yelling. After I called out a few more times, they finally quieted down. "I want to see the I.G. at Phouc Vinh," I yelled to Samuels.

No answer.

"I'm requesting an audience with the I.G. to see if a transfer was really put through. The I.G. can tell me that." I knew anyone in the military had the right to see the I.G. at any time. That request could not be refused. And, I thought the I.G. might remember me from the incident with the Enlisted Men's Club. Maybe I'd have some clout with him.

"You're going to surrender and come with us now!" Samuels blared back through the bullhorn.

"I want to see the I.G. at Phouc Vinh. If you'll take me there, I'll go with you."

"You're coming whether you want to or not. Pack your gear."

"I ain't packing shit. I said I'll go if you'll take me to Phouc Vinh but I ain't takin' my gear. After I see the I.G. I'll come back and get it if I need it."

After saying something to Bailey the sarge left for a few minutes, then returned. He yelled through the bullhorn, "We'll take you if you pack your gear before you go. You can leave it here. We'll be back to get you in fifteen minutes." They left without waiting for an answer.

I felt like I'd won a small victory and was glad to have gotten them to compromise. I got to talk a little with Java and most of the other men sat around my hooch, listening to the radio, smoking weed, and watching me pack.

"We'll guard your stuff, Treetop," they said. "They ain't gonna get away with nothin'." I began feeling more confident that things would work out. When Bailey returned, I picked up my crutches and followed him.

They flew me to Phouc Vinh, along with two other men I didn't know, but when we landed we went to the Supply Holding Office, which was nowhere near the I.G.'s office. "Wait here. They'll call you in a few minutes," the pilot said and walked outside. I sat down with the other guys who talked about their upcoming R&R.

Finally a supply sergeant I recognized from earlier visits came out and asked who wanted to see the I.G. I called out, "Right here," and hobbled into his office.

As I sat in a chair across the desk from him he said, "What can I do for you, soldier?"

"I need to talk to somebody with the Inspector General's Office," I said.

"I'm the Assistant to an Assistant I.G.," he said. "How can I help you?"

"I need to talk to the I.G. The only way you can help me is to take me to the I.G.'s office."

"The I.G.'s office is a busy place and they can't hear every pissy little complaint that comes down the pipe. That's why there are assistants like me. What do you want?"

"Listen. I know the Army regulations. Any soldier can request an audience with the I.G. That request cannot be refused. I want to see an I.G. inspector. I ain't talking to nobody else."

He leaned forward and folded his hands on the desk, looking at me like I was in the second grade. With a smirk on his face, he said, "Why don't you just tell me, soldier, and we can get this taken care of."

I looked him straight in the eye. "The only way you can help me is to let me see the I.G."

"Well, this is going nowhere," he said, standing up. "Just have a seat outside."

I went back to the waiting room, ready to sit there as long as I had to. A few minutes later a short, blond man came in and threw my gear and my M-16 in the corner, then left. *What the fuck!* It was my duffel bag—it had my name stenciled on it, along with my First Cav. patch. The guys back at the LZ were supposed to protect my stuff. *Goddamnit!* I thought. *Maybe they went back to the Psychedelic Shack after I left, not knowing they'd need to guard it.*

I was adjusting one of the bandages on my leg that was coming loose again, when all at once, the men I'd been sitting with jumped me.

"Hey!!" I yelled. "What the fuck?" I fought back with as much force as I could, but didn't have a chance. They wrestled me to the floor and held me down tight. The bandage came off my left leg and in no time at all they tied my wrists behind me with plastic tie wrap, so tight that I was sure it cut off the circulation.

Then they jerked me to my feet. "What the fuck you doing?" I yelled. "What's going on?" They didn't answer, just dragged me to a small helipad where a two-seater Bell Bubble Observer helicopter waited, took me around to the passenger side and shoved me in, with my hands still tied behind me. I saw my gear and rifle underneath my feet, but the crutches weren't there. Pushing my shoulders back, they strapped the seatbelt on me and left. When I looked over at the pilot I saw, to my horror, that it was Samuels. What was left of my rage turned to panic.

He started the rotors turning. "What's going on?" I yelled over the roaring noise. As we lifted off he looked out to his left but didn't answer. "What are you doing?" I shouted. "Where are you taking me?" My voice was shaking. My life was over. I was sure of it. We headed straight up and out over the jungle.

No answer.

"Come on, man. Tell me where we're going." I looked down, hoping to find a familiar landmark but all I could see was jungle. The guy was stone-faced, looking straight ahead. I've never been more afraid in my life. I was shaking all over, sweating, feeling like I was going to vomit. *He's going to kill me,* I thought. *Just like they'd killed Doc. Dear God in heaven,* I prayed, please *let him take me back to the LZ.*

Before long, we approached a small landing field with about a dozen tents lined up nearby. The area looked hazy, almost foggy, and I realized we were looking through a gigantic swarm of insects. We could hear their deafening hum over roar of the helicopter engine.

As we came in to land, men wrapped in poncho liners ran out to meet us, waving wildly at the millions of black bees. When the whomp, whomp of the blades stopped, the hum of the insects was unbelievably loud. The men threw poncho liners over us and someone helped me into a jeep, swatting bees all the way. They drove us to the C.O.'s tent and rushed us inside. Samuels pointed to a bench and said, "Wait there," while he went through a canvas flap into the C.O.'s office. Since the officer's area was separated from the rest of the tent only by that bit of canvas, I heard everything.

"We need to turn a soldier over to you, sir," Samuels said. "He's a troublemaker."

"I don't know why you brought the man here," a loud, deep voice answered. "I told them not to send him here."

"My C.O. approved it, sir. We can't keep him."

"I want nothing to do with this. I don't care where you take him, but he's not going to stay here. Got that soldier?"

"Yes sir. But …"

"Goddamnit," he shouted, "I said NO, soldier. Take him somewhere else. I want no part of this."

Samuels came out of the meeting red-faced and angry. Without a word, he grabbed me by the arm and jerked me to my feet, wrenching my shoulder and making the ties cut even further into my wrists. He pushed me ahead of him, then shoved me hard, and I stumbled, almost fell.

"We're outta here." he shouted to the men who had driven us in from the helipad. They covered us with poncho liners and again we ran back to the jeep, heads down, trying to avoid the bees.

Free Fall

✦

1970

They drove us back out to the helicopter and strapped me in. As they backed away, Samuels started the engine and we lifted off. "What's going on?" I yelled at him.

No response. The copter cleared the treetops.

"Where are you taking me?" I shouted.

He looked at me and shrugged. "I don't know what's going on," he shouted, in a voice that seemed to show a change of heart. "I've been trying to follow orders but they're so fucked up I don't know what they want. I'm tired of fooling with this shit. I'm just going to take you back to Phouc Vinh and turn you over to the I.G.'s office. I don't know what else to do."

I wanted to believe him. I was encouraged that he'd tried to take me to another base. He hadn't tried to kill me. I looked down at the ground about a hundred and twenty feet below us and decided that as soon as we touched down at Phouc Vinh, I'd run and hide till I could get an appointment with the I.G. I knew these men wanted to get rid of me. If I didn't get away, the next day they'd send me out on some mission in the bush and I just wouldn't come back.

I looked at Samuels. "So we're headed back to Phouc Vinh?" I asked.

He nodded, and the helicopter slowed till we were hovering high above a rice paddy. I looked down at the glare of the sun as it reflected on the acres of brown muck far below us. When I looked back to the interior of the copter, Samuels was holding a knife up to my face. I jerked back and he said, "Lean over and I'll cut off those bands."

I couldn't believe it. Relief flooded me. I wasn't going to die. I tried to lean forward but the restraint stopped me. "I can't," I said. "The seatbelt."

He unclipped it and I leaned forward, turning away from him so the plastic tie wraps were within his reach. When he cut the restraints I felt a sharp pain as the blood rushed back into my hands. When I pulled my arms around in front of me to rub my aching wrists, the copter tilted sharply starboard and Samuels shoved me out into the air. Screaming, I fell into a void. I grabbed wildly for something to hold on to, turning over and over, seeing sky, earth, sky, earth. I couldn't get my bearings. After what seemed like a very long time, I slammed into the rice paddy, landing on my side. I went completely under the water and sank into the muck, reaching around desperately, trying to determine what was up and what was down.

By some miracle I was able to stand up in the chest high water. My entire body was numb. I felt separated from myself, like I was watching someone else's life. I don't know how long I stood there, stunned. Finally I walked to a dry bank at the edge of the rice paddy. I looked up and saw the copter circling around.

My first thought was that it had been an accident and Samuels was coming back to pick me up. I waved wildly, but instead of coming down to get me, he dropped my gear and weapon, almost on top of me. Then he headed off in the distance. I couldn't make sense out of what I was seeing. I kept thinking, *Maybe he's just trying to teach me a lesson and will come back. Or maybe he needs to get help to rescue me.* I could not believe that he would leave me there.

When I became aware of a foul odor, I looked down and saw that I'd shit all over myself. The smell made me gag repeatedly, till I leaned over and vomited into the rice paddy. Then I stood back up and held my arms out from my sides, watching the copter disappear in the distance.

After some time passed, I have no idea how long, I felt my arms and legs for broken bones but found none. I took off my clothes that were covered with shit and vomit, and checked my body for leeches but didn't see any. I rinsed my shirt and pants out in the water of the rice paddy as best as I could, and put them back on. My hands were shaking so bad I could hardly get the buttons done.

Because of the jungle's canopy, the sun always set early and it was already getting dark. I wanted to stay nearby, thinking, hoping, continuing to pray that Samuels would come back. While I waited, I went through my gear and found that there were about ten rounds in a clip of ammo along with my rifle, half a canteen of water, a few stale crackers from my C-rations, and a candy bar. I had no idea how long my supplies would need to last, or where I was. But that didn't really matter because there were no battle lines; the Viet Cong were everywhere.

Before it got completely dark I went further into the jungle, listening for anything unusual. There were the sounds of birds and monkeys screeching, and the constant roar of cicadas. As I stepped on twigs and made other noises, I noticed there would be a sudden silence, but when I was quiet, the noise returned. I figured I could use that as a kind of alarm system to warn of someone approaching.

After exploring a little, I found three bushes clumped together, shaped kind of like a hut with no opening. I pulled the branches apart far enough to enter and crawled inside, dragging my gear behind me. There I hid, well camouflaged and able to see all around and above me.

I can't fully describe the blackness of the nights I spent alone, deep in the jungle. Because the canopy of trees hid the stars, there was absolutely no light at all. I held my hand in front of my face, close enough to touch my nose. Nothing. I wiggled my fingers, still nothing. I'd heard many of the night jungle sounds before, but the screeches and grunts, from what animals I could not even imagine, were terrifying. At the same time, I knew that silence could be worse. Quiet could mean something big and unexpected was moving toward me, something dangerous.

Beside the gooks, what I feared most was running into snakes, but I wouldn't have been able to see one in the dark if it slithered up right beside me. Too scared to sleep, I huddled under the bushes and prayed. My ears constantly searched for the sounds of choppers. I was petrified I might fall asleep and miss them when they came to rescue me.

My whole body was sore from being thrown from the jeep that morning, from being beaten at Phouc Vinh, and from landing in the rice paddy. My right leg ached like hell and my wrists were still swollen from the restraints. The few times I did drift off, the nightmares were so horrible that I woke myself up, screaming, covered in sweat, my skin alive with fear. If the gooks heard me, I'd be a dead man. If I was going to stay alive, I'd have to stay awake.

To keep myself alert, I tried to think of what I'd need to do to survive. Since I had no flares or any way of signaling a copter, I decided I'd have to run out by the rice paddies and wave when I heard one coming by. If I heard gooks nearby I'd stay hunkered down with my rifle ready and try not to even breathe. When I ran out of food, I'd have to find a way to trap something, but had no idea how I'd do that. I tried very hard not to think of what the gooks would do to me if they caught me. *This is what happened to Doc*, I thought. *Only he didn't make it.*

I couldn't make sense of the fact that twenty-four hours earlier I'd been sitting in my hooch, smoking dope and playing cards with Slim and Ace. How could I be out here in the jungle alone? I was in a completely different world. It didn't make sense. This couldn't be happening.

That son of a bitch, Samuels, I thought a hundred times. *When I get back I'm going to burn his ass. I still can't believe that cocksucker pushed me out of a fucking helicopter. Tried to kill me! This is a goddamned nightmare.*

For a while I'd boil with a rage so strong that every muscle in my body was taut. I felt like I might explode. My skin prickled with a frantic energy. I'd be covered with sweat and certain that any animal or person who came anywhere near me could smell me.

Later I'd sink, helpless, into a black pit of terror, shaking all over, cringing and trying not to vomit. I'd squeeze my eyes shut and pray to die.

Then I'd swing back to rage. I went back and forth, again and again. In spite of my best efforts not to, I thought about what the gooks would do to me if they found me—cut off my head and ram a bamboo stick up through my neck to set out to warn others.

I was losing my mind. I hated Samuels and all the men like him. I hated myself. I cried for my life and vowed to get revenge.

In the blackness, the strange chirping, rustling, gronking sounds made me feel like I was on another planet. If I let my imagination go I'd scare myself to death with thoughts of what might be crawling or slithering up right beside me.

Because I did my best to stay awake all night, the next morning I was exhausted. After eating a couple of crackers I drank a little water and checked out my M-16, which was in working order.

I knew the gooks would be coming back eventually to tend to the rice paddy I'd landed in the middle of, but I still decided not to move away from my spot. If Samuels or anyone else came looking for me I wanted to be where they could find me.

During the daylight I hurried out and waved at every copter I heard fly by, but nobody saw me. The hours were long and lonely. I was exhausted from lack of sleep, but didn't dare let myself doze off. The pain from my shrapnel wound was good for something; it helped me stay awake. My leg was swollen and full of pus. It ached no matter how I positioned it. I'd heard the rice paddies were fertilized with human shit and I didn't want to think about what that might mean. I tried to scrape some of the pus out with a stick but then decided I might be infecting it more. I considered pouring some of my water on it, but by noon the water was gone. I was losing hope and started thinking about where I'd go when I died. I prayed to God to save me.

Even though I was careful to ration my food, it was gone by late afternoon of the second day, and so was my hope of ever being rescued. I'd have to find my way out or starve. But if I went walking around in the jungle I could be caught and killed.

When dawn came the next morning, my entire body was stiff from hiding in the same cramped position with every muscle tensed for so long. My stomach was growling, my mouth was dry, and my leg throbbed. I knew I should be getting used to the jungle sounds around me, but I was still startled at every little thing. I wanted to get up and walk around, but I was terrified of being captured.

Around the middle of the morning I was listening for the sound of a helicopter when I heard something. Twigs breaking. The jungle sank into total silence. I grabbed my rifle and looked in the direction of the sound. *This is it,* I thought. *It's really over.*

I watched my shirt jump with each thundering beat of my heart. There was movement in the bushes about two hundred yards away. I heard voices, men talking quietly. I crouched down as low as I could. I was shaking all over. Then, I couldn't believe my ears!! The voices were speaking American English! I had to do something! I prayed silently, *Please, God. Please God. Don't let them think I'm a gook and kill me.* Then I scrambled to my feet, and still hunched over, and shouted. "Hey, G.I.! Don't shoot! I'm with the First Cav., lost from my unit."

"Who is it?" someone called. "What's your name?"

"Hairston! Private First Class Hairston, out of Phouc Vinh. I'm separated from my unit."

"Where are you? Stand up with your hands in the air."

I dropped my rifle and stood up slowly, holding my hands as high as they'd go and looked at the faces of the five best-looking men on the planet. I felt like I was in one of those scenes in the movies where the good guy is rescued. My life had been saved.

"Okay, fella. Come out here where we can see you."

I limped through the bushes, shaking all over. Tears ran down my face but I kept my arms up high in the air. "Man, am I glad to see you!"

"My God!" one of them said. "What the fuck are you doing way back in here?"

"How long you been here? Are you okay?" They gathered around me and I cried with relief, praying that this wasn't a dream.

"You got some water? Something to eat?" I asked.

"Sure, man. Name's Jackson," one of the men said. He reached out, shaking my trembling hand with one of his and steadying my wrist with his other hand. Several of the other men held their canteens out to me.

I started to gulp the water down and Jackson said, "Hey, slow down there, Brother. Take it easy, man. You don't want to make yourself sick." I stopped, knowing he was right, but I was still so thirsty. Another man looked in his C-rations and gave me three packs of peanut butter crackers. Best damn meal I ever ate.

My leg was really infected by this time and with every step I felt a sharp pain. They helped me limp along with them for almost a mile, till we reached their pickup point. Along the way they told me they were out on a reconnaissance, looking for enemy movement. I listened, but was so exhausted and glad to be rescued that I hardly knew what I was doing. When they asked how I'd gotten there, I told them what Samuels had done.

"I can't believe that fall didn't kill you," Jackson said. "You're even luckier the gooks didn't find you before we did. You're one lucky fucker."

"I guess that's one way to look at it. A lucky fucker," I said, and he laughed.

The copter met us a little after noon and it was the most beautiful bird I've ever seen. I told the pilot, "I need to go to Phouc Vinh to see the I.G. Right away."

"Okay, man," he said, "That's where we're headed anyways. What's going on?"

"Let's just say I'm at odds with my C.O." I was still shaking and crying off and on.

"Hey," he said, slapping me on the back. "No problem. We'll take you there." He reached into the pocket of his shirt and pulled out a couple of pills. "Here, take these BTs," he said. "They'll calm you down."

I swallowed the capsules without even looking at them. I'd have taken anything to help me stop shaking. We climbed aboard and the men buckled me into one of the seats. As crazy as it sounds to me now, I sat there, still trembling, still thinking to myself that somebody would be going back to look for me where Samuels had pushed me out. And I worried that they'd send me back to my LZ and the next time Samuels would kill me for sure.

Jackson sat down beside me and after we took off he said, "You need to go to the Judge Advocate General's office (JAG) instead of the I.G. The JAG's a lawyer and he can really get something done about this."

"Okay," I said. The pills had already started working and the terror was beginning to subside. "Whatever you say. Long as I get to talk to somebody."

As soon as we landed, Jackson and two of the other men went with me to file a complaint. I was way past exhausted but I knew I couldn't rest until I felt safe, and I wouldn't feel safe until I'd seen the JAG. When we got to the office I went up to the clerk and said, "I'm Eugene Hairston with A Company, First Cav. and I need to see a JAG Officer."

The guy hardly looked up. "Well, he's busy right now …"

My mind flashed back to the fall from the copter. Anger rose in my chest and it took all my self-control to keep it together. "I haven't slept in days."

"This can't wait," Jackson said, in a loud voice. "We have to see him now."

The clerk really looked at me for the first time, then stood up. "Okay, soldier. Have a seat. I'll tell him you're here."

I rubbed my forehead and pulled my hand down over my face.

He went into the office and came back out, saying, "It'll be just a few minutes." Sitting back down at the desk, he looked at me, "You okay, man?"

I nodded and Jackson and I sat down with the other two guys to wait. The next thing I remembered was "coming to," lying on the floor. Jackson and two of the other men were holding down my arms and legs.

"You okay, buddy?" Jackson asked, looking down at me.

"You all right?" someone else said.

They helped me sit up and I looked around. Desks and chairs were overturned, a typewriter was upside down on the floor and papers were scattered everywhere. A broken lamp lay by the door. "What happened?" I asked. "What happened? Who did this?"

"You did it, fella," said the clerk. "You just flipped out."

"Huh? What?" I looked up at the faces of the men around me.

One of them leaned down and said quietly, "I'm Will Tucker, the JAG. What happened, Hairston?"

"Um … I don't know, man."

"You went to sleep while you were waiting," he said, "and my clerk here, he just touched you on the shoulder to wake you up. You went completely nuts, crazy, fighting, turning over the desks and doing all this."

"Me? I did that?" I wiped my eyes and stood up. "Sorry, sir. I didn't mean to. I'm really sorry. Here, I'll clean it up."

"No, soldier, they can do it. You come in here and talk to me," Tucker said.

After I explained what had happened, Tucker stood up. "I need to go talk to some of my superiors," he said. "I want you to wait in the outer office till I come back. And," he said, smiling, and patting my shoulder, "please don't go back to sleep."

Jackson got me some strong coffee and for almost an hour we sat in the waiting room and talked to the other guys who had come with us. They were great to me; it was the only way I'd have been able to stay awake. Finally the JAG returned and called me back into his office. "All right," he said, pulling his chair up to his desk. "You can make a decision as to what you want to do here."

I had to work hard to keep my full attention on what he was saying.

"You can return to your unit and press charges against the people who tried to kill you. That's one choice. Or you can request a separation and go home. The choice is up to you, son. But I'll tell you that if you stay, I can't guarantee your safety."

"I'll be glad to leave, sir. Very glad to leave."

"I think that's probably a wise decision, Hairston. I'll have the papers drawn up under honorable conditions."

I felt anger rising in my chest. "Why wouldn't I get an Honorable Discharge? I deserve one."

"Yes, son. You do," he said, holding up his hand. "I'm just advising you what the papers will state. Shouldn't be any problem. And if there is, you just let me know and we'll get it straightened out."

"Thank you, sir," I said, taking a deep breath.

"I'll start putting the paperwork through now," he said. "Today. But it'll still take a while. Several weeks, at least."

"Yes, sir."

"Where do you want to stay during that time?"

"I want to stay with the guys who rescued me."

"Okay, soldier," he said, standing and extending his hand. "That's exactly what we'll do. And I want you to know that I'm sorry about all this."

"Thank you, sir."

"And you need to get that leg looked at."

"Yes, sir. I will. Thank you, sir."

During the month I waited on the paperwork my leg healed, and physically I felt much better. I thought about contacting Slim or Ace to let them know what had happened, but after thinking it over I figured it wouldn't be worth the risk I'd be taking. Besides, I wasn't sure what Ace would do and I didn't want him to do anything stupid.

On the Edge

◆

1970

When I got off the military plane in San Diego Air Force Base I was surprised to see people standing along chain link fences at the airfield, holding big ugly signs that read "Baby Killer" and "It's Not Our War!" and "Murderer!" I'd seen protests on television when I was on R&R, but I hadn't expected to see so many. I picked up a newspaper on my way through the airport and saw that the country's attitude toward the war in September 1970 was very different from what I remembered when I joined up in 1968. The media portrayed vets as if we were traitors, but I didn't feel like one. I wasn't ashamed of anything I'd done over there.

Walking back into my country was unreal. I was entering a completely different world. I'd spent the last nine months in a steamy jungle where the foul smell of human waste and diesel fuel was inescapable. I'd had to be aware of every little sound; ignoring the smallest noise could have cost me my life. Explosions went off at all hours of the day and night.

Back in the U.S., I was in a modern, air-conditioned airport with clean cream-colored walls and blue carpets. Noises that now sounded strange came at me from everywhere: gates moving, announcements blaring over loudspeakers, automatic sliding doors opening and closing, wheels squeaking, and people rushing around shouting. There were so many people. People everywhere. In my head I was still running on instinct, listening for anything that might mean danger.

I got through the discharge paperwork and within four hours, still wearing my Army uniform, I caught a commercial flight to cold, gray Virginia. It was strange to be with people who weren't in the military. I felt lost, disconnected from everything. I was unsure of myself, nervous, and although I knew better, I saw other people as threatening. In Vietnam, I'd learned to be careful not to let anybody ever get behind me, and seated in the middle of the plane as I was, I couldn't relax. No one said anything to me about being a soldier coming home.

In fact, the flight attendant who sold me lots of gin and tonics was the only person who spoke to me at all.

During the flight I thought about the guys I'd left behind; pictures of the hooch flashed through my head. I wondered what Ace and Slim were doing, if they were okay. I wondered if Samuels felt bad about what he had done. I was glad to be returning and could hardly wait to get home where I could feel safe.

When we got off the plane there were more protesters with the same kind of signs they'd had in San Diego. I tried to ignore them but they kept yelling and one guy even tried to spit on me. I shot him the finger and kept on walking.

I was glad to see that Bett was waiting with my mom. She'd written to me often enough, but her letters were never very personal, so I thought maybe she was just doing her duty. She ran up and gave me a big hug. I was excited to have her in my arms, but at the same time I was stunned, not sure if this was real. My mom was standing a little distance away and when I walked over to her she smiled and patted me on the arm. "Glad you made it home," she said. "You're skinny as a pole. We'll have to fatten you up."

I reached down to hug her but she turned away.

"I'm fixing your favorite supper soon as we get home," she said.

"That sounds good, Mom," I said.

Bett hung on my arm. "Oh, Billy," she said. "I'm so glad you're back. I've got so much to tell you."

"I'm glad to be back, too," I said, trying hard to act as if everything around me seemed normal. When we got to the baggage area, I gave Bett a long kiss and smelled the liquor on her breath. That surprised me. That was new.

As we walked to my mom's car, Bett said, "I thought we'd go out tonight."

"Oh, I don't know," I said, my stomach giving a lurch. "Tonight?" I needed to be away from people, to be all alone, all alone in a safe place. Or just with Bett. The thought of being in some loud nightclub filled me with dread.

"Sure," she said. "I talked to Buck and J.J., and they said to meet them at this new club in town."

"Okay," I said, not wanting to disappoint her. *Oh well,* I thought, *if Buck's going to be there I'll be okay.* "That's cool, I guess."

I got in the back seat of the car and as Bett slid in next to me, she leaned over and whispered, "I'm not wearing any panties." I smiled at her and thought to myself that she changed a lot while I was gone. She would never have said anything like that before. She was louder and her dress was definitely tighter than her dad used to allow. And there was alcohol on her breath.

On the drive home she talked about everybody she knew. "Janet's been going out with Bookie again, even after he left her for that slut, Danielle."

"Hmmm," I said.

"Yeah, and Archie's been working at the shipyard and got promoted to supervisor. He's really making something of himself. He's been talking about going back to school."

"Cool."

"Racine and Claude got married and had twin girls that her mama watches while they both work."

I tried to pay attention, to say the right thing in response to her, but it was so hard to focus. I didn't care about any of it.

At one point she turned to me and asked, "What was it like over there, Billy?" When I didn't answer, she just stared at me, then said, "Oh never mind, Baby. We can talk about that later."

As we walked into the house, my mom said, "I got your room all made up for you, Billy. Take your stuff in and get unpacked while I fix your dinner. Bett can help me here for a few minutes."

"Okay," I said, heading to my bedroom with my duffel bag. I threw it on the bed and looked around. Everything was just as I'd left it, green walls, green and blue linoleum tiles on the floor, a bare light bulb in the ceiling, and a dark green overstuffed chair in the corner. The same white curtains hung at the window and the table scarf on the dresser was the same one that had been there since I was a kid. After Vietnam the room seemed very bright and clean.

Ivy, my younger half-sister, ran up behind me. "Hey, Billy Junior," she said. "Welcome home." She gave me a quick hug, then headed out the door. "I'm going to the movies. Maybe I'll talk to you later." She was gone.

As I put my clothes in the dresser, images flashed through my mind: the faces of the protesters on the tarmac as I got off the plane, flaming napalm, the constant booming sounds of explosions, Maya, the papasan's black teeth, Samuels, Ace smiling at me from the lawn chair near our hooch. Pictures kept marching before me like a movie. My eyes filled with tears. I sat down on the bed and held my head in my hands, determined not to cry. If I started, I wouldn't be able to stop. *I'm home now,* I told myself. *Everything's going to be all right,* although I couldn't see how anything would ever be all right again.

I heard footsteps. I wiped my eyes and looked up as Bett came in and stood in front of me. "Hey," I said, "There's something I want to show you."

I was surprised when she moved in between my legs and shoved the duffel bag to the floor. We fell back on the bed as she pressed her body hard against mine and kissed me. "And what's that you want me to see?" she asked with a sexy smile, wiggling against me.

"This is something we did in Vietnam. We call it 'giving Dap,'" I said, pushing her back as I stood up. "Look at this." I pulled her to her feet and held my right palm up to her. "Here, put your hand up here …" I showed her how to "give Dap," and when she'd learned to do it, she grabbed my hand and pulled me close.

The kiss was hard and deep, and we fell back on the bed, tearing at each other's clothes. She slid on top of me, wildly kissing my face, my neck, down my chest. When I finally entered her, she came with loud, panting wails, and I came right with her. For the first time since I'd left home almost two years before, things felt better.

Later, we got up and I showered and dressed in my street clothes. As we walked downstairs I smelled fried chicken, French fries and baked beans, my favorites. When we sat down at the kitchen table, my mom pulled homemade biscuits out of the oven.

"All your favorites, Billy Junior. Here's some biscuits," she said, putting two on my plate and sliding the butter dish over. "Bett, we got plenty, here. You eat all you want." Then she took a beer and went to the living room where I heard the television click on.

I forced myself to take a few bites, but that was the best I could do. Buck called about 9:00. "Hey, Bro," he said, "just want to say welcome back to the world. J.J. and me, we're gonna save you two seats at the table tonight. Meet us at ten."

The nightclub was dark, loud, and smoky, nothing I hadn't been used to a couple of years ago, but now I was instantly afraid, on alert. The talking, the music, unexpected movements all set me spinning down a deep dark hole. I was terrified, but I knew I couldn't show it. Not now. I had to be tough. If I didn't act tough, I'd be a victim.

They were waiting for us at a table near the door. "Welcome, Brother," Buck said, standing up and giving me a long hug. "Hey, man, gimme some Dap."

"What's Dap?" J.J. asked, watching us.

"We'll teach you," Buck said. "It's something we learned in Vietnam."

Buck and J.J. looked the same as they always had, but that was on the outside. Because Buck and I had both been to Vietnam we had a common bond; we'd been through things J.J. and the others knew nothing about. Buck had joined up a year or so before me and nearly died after he was sprayed with machine gun bullets. He'd told me that his scars were in a straight line from his right shoulder to his left thigh and he'd spent a year in a hospital before coming home. I knew he understood what I was going through.

Several brothers I went to high school with came over. "Hey, Billy Junior," one of them said. "Did you kick some ass over there?"

Another said, "Glad you made it back, Bro. Did you kill any V.C.?"

I shook their hands and said, "Hey, man. Good to see you." I just wanted to be alone.

"Looks like you lost some weight. Guess Bett'll fix that."

"He's a mean, lean fighting machine," Buck said, giving me Dap again.

Another brother came over and put out his hand. "Well, the hero's home. Why ain't you wearing your uniform? Got your gun with you?"

"Good to see you, man," I said, forcing myself to look him in the eye and smile. It took every ounce of my self-control.

After we finished our drinks, J.J. went to get us another round. He'd just left when a guy came over and sat down in his chair. "Hey, Billy Junior, welcome home," he said. "Kill any babies over there?"

I couldn't place him but figured he must be somebody I went to school with.

"Must have been rough," he said. "I heard a few stories. Heard them little tiny gooks are real killers." As he went on talking I noticed that his words were directed to me, but his eyes kept going to Bett. I tried to ignore it, and when J.J. came back with the drinks, the guy left.

I took a sip of the cold beer and asked Bett, "Who was that? I don't remember him."

"Oh, sure," she said. "He went to high school with us. We call him Blow."

"Why'd he come over here?"

"I don't know, Baby. Just wanted to welcome you home, I guess." She kissed me on the neck. "I'm so glad you're back."

"Ain't his daddy that big gambler? The one with lots of money?"

"Oh, yeah, I think so. I'm not sure," she said, standing up. "Listen, Baby, I'm gonna go cut in on this dance. I'll be right back."

Bett was a little drunk when I took her home. She'd sure changed; she hardly drank at all before, but I liked the new Bett. And she'd made it clear she liked me. Her dad didn't want me calling her at their house, she said, but she promised to call me the following day.

The next morning I lay in bed remembering how it was before I went to Vietnam. How I'd get all dressed up to go out partying with my buddies and come home so stoned I could hardly make it in the front door. I recalled the few girls I'd made love to, the high school basketball games I'd played in, the fights with my mom over my grades. It felt like another lifetime … or like some other man's life. When I'd left Portsmouth, I'd been able to sleep all night. No one had ever tried to kill me. My biggest problem had been when my mom wouldn't let me in the house because I'd missed my curfew.

I remembered those things. But I felt nothing. I wondered why I was so numb.

When I got out of bed and went into the kitchen, the feeling of disorientation continued. It was like I was in someone else's skin. In the days that followed I couldn't relax or feel anything even close to normal. Things that used to be ordinary, like the sounds of trucks roaring down the street, neighbors yelling, doors slamming, the stink of the soap factory down the street when they burned their waste; they all sent me back to Vietnam. My brain was running constantly. I couldn't stop.

And I didn't hear from Bett for three days. Then late one night, I was lying in bed with a fifth of bourbon determined to drink myself numb when there was a knock on the door. It was Bett. I didn't know whether to be happy or not. She followed me into the living room and sat beside me on the couch.

"Where you been?" I asked. "Why haven't you called me?"

"I just needed to talk to some people, Baby. Just to get a few things straight," she said snuggling up close. "You know you been gone a long time, and I ain't just been sitting around here doing nothing." She put her hand on my knee, cocked her head and looked up at me. "You know I love you, baby. You're the one for me."

I turned to her. She was so beautiful, and she'd said she loved me. I wanted to believe her. I reached for her hand. "Come over here to me, you sweet thing. Let's go get busy for a while."

When we stood up, she hugged me around the neck with one hand and slipped the other hand down the front of my pants. "I told my mom I'm staying at a girlfriend's," she said. "I'm gonna be here with you all night. And I'm gonna love you all over, Baby. Like you never had it before."

◆   ◆   ◆

About three in the morning, Bett's screaming woke me up. "Billy Junior!! Stop!! What's wrong with you? You gone crazy?"

When I opened my eyes, I was straddling her on the bed with my hands around her throat, and she was hitting me as hard as she could. As soon as I let go, she scrambled away. She stopped at the door and flipped the light on.

"Billy, what the fuck is wrong with you?" she yelled.

I moved to the side of the bed and held my head in my shaking hands. I was covered in sweat. I waited before I spoke, afraid I'd done something unforgivable. "I don't know what the hell happened. I guess I was dreaming. I'm sorry Baby, I'm so sorry. I don't know ..."

"Are you crazy?"

"I don't know. Maybe I am," I said, looking at her beautiful naked body. "I'd never hurt you on purpose, you know that."

"I just touched your arm," she said. "You were rolling around and shaking your head back and forth, yelling like somebody was after you."

"I'm really sorry." I stood up and moved toward her and although I could still see fear in her eyes, she let me put my arms around her and hold her. "From now on, if I ever do that again, don't touch me. Don't even get near me. Just let me go through it."

"Okay, Baby," she said, relaxing. "You're home now. It's okay. You're safe."

◆   ◆   ◆

The only way I could avoid the nightmares was to stay awake, so I did everything I could to keep from falling asleep. The method that seemed to work best was to get high or doped up and let my imagination go to situations where I was in charge, where I was the hero. When I had dreams about being shoved out of the helicopter, I woke up screaming; I was covered in sweat; completely, totally, absolutely consumed by fear. I didn't think I could keep on living if I had to go through it again. I'd always known I couldn't trust other people. Now I couldn't even trust myself.

Although the months I spent in Vietnam were filled with pain and horror, it was also the first time in my life I'd ever felt really close to people, like I was part of a family. That became more and more clear to me after I got home. Over there my friends joked to be funny instead of trying to hurt me. I'd learned to trust them. We'd watched each other's backs and depended on each other for survival. During the nights on guard duty, sometimes huddling in bunkers while incoming mortars exploded around us, we'd shared our secrets. We'd laughed together and cried together. We'd talked about each other's relatives till I felt like I was part of a huge family. We'd loved each other like brothers.

When I came back home and left them all behind, I was totally isolated and alone. It was hard to face the fact that I'd probably never see any of my buddies again, men I'd grown to love and to trust. And nobody wanted to hear about

them. My affection for them was colored by the anti-war protests and name-call-
ing, and my pride in their actions seemed tarnished. My family and friends
thought I was more concerned about my Army buddies than I was about them.
"We don't care about a bunch of losers," they said. "You're back here now. Get
with it."

At first, my old friends bought me drinks and dope and I talked a little about
what I'd seen and done, about the differences between the Americans and Vietnamese. But a lot of them only wanted to hear war stories about the gore and the
horror, the things that I wanted to forget because they brought back memories,
and memories brought nightmares.

One night I was out drinking with Will and Mackie, a couple of guys I knew
from high school.

"I don't know why you went to Vietnam," Will said. "That was whacked."

At first I argued, "Come on, man. We were there to help those people. The
commies were trying to take over."

"That's a bunch of shit. It was nothing but a political thing," said Mackie.
"You're stupid for going over there."

"You don't know what you're talking about," I said. "We put our lives on the
line to help those people. Some of my friends died over there."

"And they died for nothing, man," Will said, slamming his fist on the table.
"If they'd been smart enough, they wouldn't have died. They should'a used their
heads."

"That just ain't so," I said.

"Aw, if I'd been there, I could have gotten myself out of anything," Mackie
said. "You just got to keep a cool head. Ain't no problem for me. Just stay alert
and be able to hit your target."

"And another thing," said Will, "dropping that napalm, that's just the coward's way out. Any man with real guts could stand his ground and fight man-to-
man. Only a coward would run away." The more my friends talked, the quieter I
got.

Most people didn't believe me when I talked about some of the things I'd seen
and been through. Although I trusted Aunt Lena more than anyone, when I visited her, I didn't talk to her about it. I knew she'd just tell me that I had to trust
God to take care of me. Even Bett said, "That couldn't have happened. The
Army wouldn't let somebody push you out of a helicopter." Buck was the only
one who understood, and we didn't even have to talk about it to know we were
supporting each other.

Even after I'd been home for several months, the constant awareness of my surroundings, the vigilance that had kept me alive, was still second nature. I couldn't let go of that mind-set. When I walked into a room I automatically checked out every exit. I always sat near the door—never with my back to an open area. I couldn't stand being in crowds or standing too close to people. If anyone came up to me unexpectedly, I had an immediate reflex that jolted me into a defensive mode, ready to protect myself.

Being engulfed in darkness scared me, and my immediate reaction was to go toward the light. But when I was in the light, I could be seen and others could attack me. I couldn't wear headphones to listen to music because I wouldn't be able to hear someone approaching.

To escape the constant, intolerable, uncontrollable need to be alert at all times, I used intravenous heroin to relax. Then I needed cocaine to get me up and moving; and, of course, I never stopped using marijuana and alcohol. Basically, I did anything that would take me out of me, to escape the fear and desperation deep inside. There was nothing but fear and pain. Fear and pain.

When I was high on heroin, I had a sense of being present in the world while having no concerns about anything, a state of deep relaxation where I was aware of the people around me, but for that small space of time, I had no fear about what might happen next. In addition, it made sex hotter and I lasted longer. What more could anyone want?

Good Intentions

✦

1970

After I'd been home a few weeks I tried to call Columbia Yachts, where I'd worked after school before I joined the service, hoping to get my old job back. When I learned they'd gone out of business, I realized that meant I was eligible for unemployment so I went and applied for it the same day. The Employment Office was a busy place, people waiting everywhere, telephones ringing and typewriters clacking from the cubicles behind the receptionist. I signed in, took a plastic number card hanging from a small stand, and sat down.

The people waiting, for the most part, looked like they were down and out, and having to sit there an hour or two did nothing to improve anyone's mood. More than once I heard raised voices, "I told you, I been to that fucking place twice already. They told me not to come back," or "This ain't enough to feed my babies I got at home. What you expect me to do?"

I went back to the office every week or so and each time they sent me to apply for two or three minimum wage jobs. I filled out applications all over town but couldn't get hired. Like all ex-servicemen, I had to present the Military's DD-214 Form with my application, which verified my time in the service. Under the Reason for Discharge, my Code Number was SPN-264, which, at the time, I really hadn't noticed. If I'd known that those numbers indicated I had what we now call Post Traumatic Stress Disorder (PTSD) and that I'd used drugs, I might have understood why no one would hire me. I still find it hard to believe that the military would inform the business world of my problems, but offer no help to me or the other veterans who were in the same condition.

I've heard that PTSD was first documented during the Civil War under names like Battle Fatigue or Shell Shock. Since that time, Army units were usually kept together from basic training till they returned home, which gave tremendous support to the troops. Because the war in Vietnam was never officially declared a war, that did not happen for Vietnam vets.

◆   ◆   ◆

One day, as I was into my second hour of waiting in the Employment Office, a brother in his twenties, wearing a brown leather jacket and combat boots, sat down next to me. He looked at my Army jacket and said, "Big Red 1."

"First Cav.," I answered, and he held up his hand and gave me Dap.

"Baxter," he said. "Baxter Fulton. Bax."

"Billy Hairston," I said. "They call me Tree."

"This fucking world sucks," he said. "I risk my life fighting for my country and when I get home I can't get a job digging ditches. 'Cause I ain't got no experience."

"You're right, Brother," I answered.

"I was a tank pilot," he said. "Man, I ran a fifty thousand dollar piece of equipment, but I ain't good enough to operate a three hundred dollar dishwashing machine."

"Hey, Bro. I know what you're going through. I was a dispatcher. Men's lives depended on me every fucking day. But I ain't good enough to fry burgers."

"Hey, listen," he said, "there's a hangout where brothers meet in a church over in Chesapeake. It's a place for Vietnam vets to support each other and they got a crazy black library. You might want to check it out."

That sounded great. "I'm down," I said. "And I just got me a car, so I can get there." For the first time in a while, something sounded hopeful. Bett's cousin, Lee, was a stocky dark-skinned man who smiled a lot and made good money driving a city dumpster truck. Not long after I got home, he'd given me a 1964 Mustang that he'd patched up. It had "I Will Be There" written in black on the driver's side rear door and I took a lot of ribbing about that, because the car was always breaking down and often I didn't "get there."

The next day I followed Bax's directions and drove to the church in Chesapeake, about an hour away. It was an old ivy-covered gray stone building with stained glass windows and a courtyard. I talked to a brother there who told me about Black Brothers United (BBU), which was created by Vietnam vets who wanted to make a difference in the black community. "You want to be down with the group?" he asked.

"Sure, man. I'm down like ground round," I said.

Although I never did see Bax there, I drove to the church almost every day for weeks. I'd hoped that since they were vets, I might make friendships like I had with the guys in Vietnam, because we'd been through a lot of the same things.

While that didn't happen, the men at the BBU actually believed that by working together we could make a difference in the world, and that gave me hope. "Together we stand, divided we fall," they'd say. "Let's take back our neighborhoods from the white politicians."

We met in the big, musty church basement where books lined the walls and there was more information about black writers and inventors than I'd ever seen. I'd sit myself down in one of the big overstuffed chairs next to a lamp, and read through the winter afternoons. I even wrote a little myself.

I learned that George Washington Carver was a chemist who invented peanut butter and lots of ways to use other plants. Thomas Jennings invented dry cleaning. Dr. Charles Drew came up with the idea of having blood banks and started them up all over the world. A doctor named Daniel Williams performed the first open heart surgery, Garrett Morgan invented the first traffic light. The list went on and on and on. All these people I'd never heard anything about gave me a new pride in my race.

The BBU held rallies where we talked about black pride and black power. We planned food drives and debated how to build up our neighborhoods. We wanted to get the hoodlums and drug dealers off the street corners, arrange transportation for the elderly to do their grocery shopping, and clean up the whole area. We mowed lawns and helped people paint and fix their places up in return for a meal or two.

We had good intentions, but we couldn't find the money to support our ideas. Our fundraisers weren't bringing in much, so we tried a different approach. We decided to rob the rich and give to the poor. We started breaking into grocery stores owned by whites, selling everything we stole at half price, and putting the money in the bank to go toward our projects.

Most of us still couldn't find work and so we had plenty of time to put into getting organized, but when things didn't go smoothly we lost our determination to make a difference. No one ever brought drugs or alcohol to the meetings out of respect for the church, but one day that all changed. We were in the basement and one of the brothers brought in a joint that was the size we used to roll in Vietnam. "Hey, man, remember these days?" he said. Well, we remembered those days real well.

As we grew more discouraged, we shared our feelings of self-pity, anger and defeat. Eventually we decided we needed the money we had in the bank for ourselves. It wasn't long after that we just met to get high and our plans were tossed out the window. So, to sum it all up, first we stole to support our neighborhoods, then to support ourselves, then to support our drug habits. In the end we even sold drugs in the very neighborhoods we'd wanted to clean up.

I was unhappy with the changes in the BBU, but I stayed active anyway. My need to be a part of the group was more important than following my own conscience. I was lucky enough not to get caught when we finally got raided by the police, and the organization was shut down. But by then my career as a criminal was well underway.

When I look back on that part of my life, I now see that I'd become an actor and played whatever parts I thought would make people like me. I seldom voiced my own opinions, and if a confrontation started after I'd said something, I ended up agreeing with the other side. Gradually I became isolated, a very confused, angry young black man. I continued to do anything I could think of to stay awake twenty-four/seven, to escape the never-ending, terrifying nightmares. I was a drug addict, full of explosive energy, completely unable to sit still. No matter how much effort I put into calming down, one of my legs or my hands were constantly jiggling.

◆   ◆   ◆

One night in November I was watching The Ed Sullivan Show in my bedroom when Bett came stomping in. She flipped off the television and said, "I'm through with all this shit at home." Holding up her hand, she counted off her fingers, "My mother, my father, my sister. They all suck." She dropped down on the bed beside me. "My father gave me a 9:00 curfew and he won't let me drive the car. My mother's always crying and wringing her hands about what a sinner I am and how God's gonna punish me. And Bonita don't never do a damn thing wrong. She's the good daughter and I'm the bad one. I hate them all and want to get the fuck outta there." She snuggled up and kissed me hard.

"Do you love me?" she asked.

"Uh … yeah, sure," I answered. "I love you."

"Then let's get married," she said, pulling me close. "I want to be Mrs. Billy Hairston. Then my mom and dad can't tell me what to do."

I sat up and looked at her. "You kidding me?" I said. "I ain't got no job, no money, or even my own place."

"That's all right, Baby," she said, kissing my neck and slipping her hand under my shirt. "I got some money and I can call Lee. He'll help us."

"You think this is a good idea? Right now? I don't know …"

"Yes, Baby. This is the perfect time."

I knew this probably wasn't the right thing to do, but I didn't want to lose her. So, I said, "Well, okay. I guess so."

"Tomorrow? We can go to Carolina tomorrow. If we're there by noon we can be back by late afternoon. I'll get Lee to drive us."

What the hell, I thought. "I'm down with it," I said. "Let's do it."

When she returned from making the phone call, she said, "Lee's gonna pick us up early in the morning." With a big smile, Bett pushed me back on the bed and sat astride me, reaching down to unzip my pants. "I can hardly wait!" she said. "Mrs. Bett Hairston."

"That's cool," I said, pulling her blouse off over her head. "You gonna stay here tonight." She wriggled out of her panties as I pulled her close.

Later I found my mom in the kitchen, washing the dishes. I smelled a pie baking in the oven. I sat down at the table and said, "Just want you to know that Bett and me, we been talking about getting married."

She rinsed a dish and put it in the drainer, but didn't look up.

"She's the only girl who's stuck with me," I said to her back. "I think it'll be a good thing. Help me settle down."

She shook her head and turned around to face me, grabbing a towel and wiping her hands. She threw the cloth on the counter and said, "You got no job, no place to live, no way to take care of a family. You ain't got a pot to piss in, nothing but the clothes on your back." She shook her finger in my face. "I don't know where you're staying but you ain't staying here."

"Just wanted to let you know. We're getting married tomorrow."

She glared at me, took one of her Regent beers out of the refrigerator and walked out of the kitchen. I sat there for a few minutes, wondering why I'd ever expect anything but that sort of answer, then went back upstairs.

Bett jumped up when I got to the room and asked, "What did she say? What did she say?"

"She's okay with it," I answered.

◆   ◆   ◆

It was freezing the next morning when Lee pulled up out front and honked the horn. I picked up a paper bag that held a fifth of gin and a six-pack of beer for the trip; we went out and climbed in the car. Although I'd brought enough to share, I was the only one who drank. And I drank all the way there. We bought the license, got the blood test, and found a Justice of the Peace all in the same building. By 1:00 we were married. And I sat in the back seat alone and drank all the way home.

When we pulled up at Bett's house that afternoon I asked, "Which one of us is gonna tell your parents?"

Bett looked at me. "We can do it together."

"I'm waiting right here," Lee said. "Hope nobody gets killed."

As we walked up to Bett's front door, I dreaded what lay ahead. Bett had given them so much trouble lately my only hope was that they'd be relieved to have her move out. We stopped outside the door and I kissed her.

She said, "I'm gonna say it right off. Get it over with." As she opened the door and we stepped inside she called out, "Mom! Dad! Billy and me got married!"

Her dad was sitting in their comfortable middle-class living room in his comfortable, middle-class armchair, watching the news. Her mom came in from the kitchen, her hands on her hips. I walked over to her dad, trying to look confident, and put out my hand. He did not reach up to shake it. I said, "Sir, I really love your daughter and I'm gonna do my best to take care of her and protect her. I want to make you proud of me."

He didn't move at first, then a look of defeat crossed his face. He got up and turned off the TV. Her mother started crying.

"Bett," she yelled. "What have you done? You've ruined your life. You're only nineteen. You don't know what you're doing." She put her hands to her face and started sobbing.

Bett went over to hug her, but her mom held her hands up and backed away. "Mama," she said. "I love him. He's my man. And he's a good man."

"Oh, Bett," her mom said. "You're supposed to finish college. You'll never finish now."

"Yes, I will, Mama," Bett said. "We talked all about it. Billy's gonna get a job and support me so I can finish school. He promised."

That was the first I'd heard of that.

"Yes, ma'am," I said. "I'm a veteran, and we're supposed to get preference when it comes to getting hired." I didn't tell them I hadn't been able to find any real work since I got home.

Then her dad spoke up. "Follow me, Billy," he said, walking toward the kitchen. "I have a few things to say to you." He told me to sit down at the table and he stood in front of me, his arms crossed.

"Young man, you and my daughter have ignored everything I've said. I don't care if you are a veteran; that doesn't mean you'll be able to take care of Bett.

From what I've heard you're a drug addict and can't even support yourself. You still live with your mother."

I wanted to defend myself but everything he said was true. The familiar feelings of shame and worthlessness closed in on me.

"You're drunk right now. You smell like a barroom." He looked at me with disgust. I knew he wanted to hit me and I leaned back.

"I truly love Bett," I said, "and I want to do right by her."

"Well, seems she's chosen to make her bed; now she's gonna have to lie in it. I want you to know that once you take her out of this house, she's your responsibility. I won't be helping either one of you."

"Yes, sir," I said. "I understand." But in the back of my mind I thought, *I'll make Bett happy. I'll prove him wrong.*

Her dad shook his head and went back into the living room. I followed him and when Bett saw me, she took my hand and led me back out to the car.

"Well, you're both still alive," Lee said. "That's something."

When Lee dropped us off at my Mom's, she was at the kitchen table, drinking a beer and reading the Bible. We sat down with her, but I stayed quiet while Bett did the talking. No point in my saying anything.

"You know he ain't got no job," my mom said.

"I know," Bett answered.

"Ain't got his own place. Ain't got a pot to piss in."

"I know."

I outlined one of the flowers on the oilcloth that covered the table and tried not to let my mom's comments bother me.

"That boy, he's no good, like his daddy."

"I know," Bett said. "But I love him. I'm in college and you just watch. We're both gonna get good jobs."

"Oh, yeah," my mom said.

"Right now, we just need a place to live for a little while. If you'll let us stay with you, it won't be for long, you'll see."

My mom was silent for what seemed like a very long time. Then she stood up and pushed her chair under the kitchen table. "Counting Ivy, that's gonna put four of us in this little place what can hardly hold three." She paused. "I guess you can stay, but just till you get on your feet. Then you got to get out."

"Oh, thank you," Bett called after her, as my mom walked into the living room and clicked on the TV. "You won't be sorry."

Later that night Bett asked me, "Why does your mama always say your daddy's no good? He's a big shot, I hear. What's wrong with that?"

"I don't know," I answered. "She's always hated him. But then, I always heard he'd got himself a reputation as a ladies' man, so that might be why."

Two days later Bett moved all her belongings to my mom's two-bedroom apartment in the projects. And thus began the family of the Billy Hairstons.

Bett kept the house clean and cooked good meals so my mom was happy. We never heard from Bett's mom and dad, but one day Bonita came over to visit her sister. I stood in the hall where they couldn't see me and listened to them talk.

"Mom and Daddy both hate that you've done this," Bonita said. "Daddy says you gonna be sorry if you ain't already. Billy ain't no good."

"I know, I know," Bett answered. "But I'm out of the house. Ain't nobody telling me how to run my life. I'll show them!"

"You're gonna end up with nothin'. Billy's just gonna buy dope with every penny that comes in. Ain't gonna be no money for you to finish school. Daddy ain't gonna help now you married."

"You just mind your own fuckin' business," Bett said, raising her voice.

"You gonna be living with Billy and his mama till you're an old lady."

After going at it for a few minutes, they forgot they were mad and went out shopping together. That was one thing I envied, their ability to argue with each other and then be friends again a few minutes later. I didn't know how to do that.

◆   ◆   ◆

As the weeks went by, I tried to do the right thing, to get steady work and take care of Bett. It was crowded with four of us in the small apartment and it was often tense. I loved Bett, truly loved her, but more and more, drugs and drink came first. When I tried to go without using, I walked into a dark prison of hopelessness. I was anxious and angry, short-tempered and consumed with fear. The thought of using never left me. Nothing mattered except getting rid of that awful feeling.

The only jobs I was able to get paid minimum wage, and though I always got "atta-boys" from my bosses I never stayed anywhere long enough to get promoted. I always got high before making any plans, so when I decided whether to keep a job or leave it, the decision was made under the influence of drugs or alcohol. I complained about the world and how unfair everything was, and then got high to escape.

I now know that as a drunk and an addict, I was an embarrassment to my family and friends, but back then I saw myself as a fun guy, getting high and acting the fool. I was never a threatening drunk, I'd just do stupid things like putting catsup in my coffee at a restaurant and calling the waitress over to complain. Seemed to me that getting smashed and throwing up on people was just my way of showing what a comic I was. Although I was always laughing, it was just to cover up the fear and pain, and the horror of the nightmares that always haunted me.

It was almost a year after we got married that Bett and I were finally able to move into our own place, a little two-bedroom house in the Douglas Park Housing Units. It was great to finally be on our own, but we didn't have much to start out with: a couch, a table, a TV, a stereo, and a bed; but it was ours. I promised Bett that we'd soon be able to buy new furniture, and my intentions were always good, but we both knew that would probably never happen. By then, Bett had dropped out of school and was working at the Holiday Inn as a maid. I was hustling and taking the only jobs I could find, which turned out to be part-time.

Bett's father was true to his word. The only time she asked him for money, he said no and told her not to ever ask again. Bonita still wanted to hang out with Bett, but she hated me. If I walked into a room, she walked out.

Bett didn't complain about my drugs at first, but my "I don't give a damn" attitude forced her to take over all the household responsibilities. Gradually she developed an "I don't give a damn" attitude towards me and started seeing other men. "Since I'm taking care of the bills," she'd say, "I'll do whatever I want, and you can go get high and fuck yourself." Our life together became a vicious cycle. The worse I got into drugs the more Bett partied, which in turn depressed me so I sought more escape through drugs and alcohol.

One Saturday night I was lying on the sofa, smoking reefer when Bett walked in from the bedroom wearing a new red dress. She stood in front of the mirror, combing her hair and I said, "Where you going to?"

"To play cards."

"Why you got to do that?" I was pissed. She never stayed home with me.

She turned around and put her hands on her hips, just like her mother. "You don't pay the bills. Somebody's got to make some money around here. You sure ain't doing it."

I leaned forward on the couch and reached for her, but she moved away. "Why don't you just stay home tonight, Baby?" I said. "You know I can't go to those parties. Too many people. All that noise, everybody in my face. You know it makes me crazy. I can't do it."

"Yes, you could. If you really wanted to," she said, stepping into her shoes. "If you'd get off those fucking drugs."

"I want you to stay here with me."

"I'll be back in a couple of hours," she said, slamming the door behind her.

At three in the morning I heard her come into the bedroom. While she was taking off her clothes, I turned over and said, "You playing cards all this time?"

"Yeah," she said, sitting on the side of the bed.

"I know you ain't been playing all night. Who was you with?"

"I wasn't with nobody. You know, if you'd stop getting high all the time I wouldn't have to go out."

I sat up. "There was other men there, playing cards. I know there was."

Bett lay down on the bed, facing away from me. "Go to sleep."

I knew she'd been with somebody, I could tell by the way she talked and the way she smelled. But I couldn't think of anything I could do about it. I couldn't get out of the awful cycle I was in. Everything was completely out of control.

◆   ◆   ◆

My life with Bett got worse and worse. I was a drunk and an addict, always pointing my finger at the world and acting like it was everyone else's fault, never mine. But inside, I always knew I was irresponsible. Secretly, I wanted something to magically take me out of the ghetto. I daydreamed that miracles could really happen. Other times I prayed that God would take me away, and I'd imagine how sad everybody would be, standing around my casket saying, "You brothers know he really was a good man underneath it all."

Drugs ran my life. I did whatever I needed to do to get money. Heroin still helped the most because it gave me the calmness and detachment from the world that I craved. Without heroin I was paranoid all the time. I thought constantly about Bett partying with those other men and felt very sorry for myself. So I used more …

When I ran out of drug money I hustled small items, nothing big. Usually, I'd go into a convenience store that kept cigarettes under the counter, wait till the cashier was helping somebody at a different register, and reach over and pull out five packs at a time. Lots of times the other customers saw what I was doing but only once did a man say, "Hey, that's not right. You need to put those back." But I just walked out of the store. After two hits, I'd have ten packs, a carton of cigarettes to sell. Or I'd steal cans of Spam or corned beef, or sometimes even clothes, then sell them for half the original price.

When I got caught shoplifting, I'd hope that the judge would be lenient with me and let me off, and almost before that thought was out of my head I'd pray that he'd put me in prison and throw away the key. I'd plan my suicide, then fifteen minutes later dream of finding something that would take me out of the slums and turn my life around. In reality, I had no idea at all how to control my behavior.

As I got more and more depressed, my attitude changed. Instead of not taking responsibility for anything I did, I blamed myself for everything that was wrong. I couldn't find any way out. We lost the house in Douglas Park and Bett moved back with her parents. I was living with my mom and my sister again. We all argued constantly. I had no peace. There was nothing positive in my life.

One night, after another fight with Bett, I decided I couldn't go on living. Everything hurt too much. The only aim I had in life was to get more drugs to take away the pain. When I decided to kill myself, I felt hopeful for the first time in months. There was a solution to my problem after all, a way to end the twisting, unremitting pain. I bought twenty valiums off the street with my last little bit of money, went straight home and downed them with two Colt 45s. I curled up on my bed and thought about how much better off everybody would be without me, and how they'd regret the way they'd treated me.

I woke in a bright emergency room, staring up at strangers dressed in white, all talking at once. I told the doctor that I couldn't see any point in going on living, and he pumped my stomach and sent me home with my mother.

For a week after that I left the house only long enough to get some drugs, then returned home and stayed in bed. I ate nothing, slept only when I passed out.

The need to make money to buy drugs eventually drove me back out to find work. Several weeks after the suicide attempt, a friend helped me get hired on at the naval yard. The contracts for jobs there lasted only a few months, at which time you'd sign a new contract or you were out of work. My main job was a nasty one, but I was there every day. I cleaned the sludge out of the ships' oil tanks, which meant climbing down into the fuel reservoir, hosing it down, brushing it out, and hauling away the sludge that was left. It was toxic, slimy, dangerous work. Men routinely passed out and fell off the ladders, and we had to haul them out.

After several months I applied for an opening for one of the supervisory positions but instead of hiring me, the area manager gave the job to his son. "That ain't fair!" I said to anybody who would listen. "I'm a damned veteran and I need a break! I'm filing a protest!" In the end, my attitude cost me my job. When my contract expired they chose not to renew it. Out of work again, I went back to hustling.

Empty Chambers

◆

1970–1971

My first burglary arrest was a midnight job with "Pop," an older man who was kind of the head criminal in the neighborhood, and one other guy. I was proud that Pop chose me to go on the heist and was determined to show no fear. This was a big deal. I'd be one of the really tough guys.

It was about 2 a.m. when we removed a big exhaust fan from the back of a Pep Boy's Auto Supply store and the other guy and I climbed in. We grabbed anything that had an electric cord and handed the take to Pop, who waited in the dark cluttered alleyway outside. He put the loot in his trunk and came back for more.

Finally, Pop called in to us, "That's it. We gotta go." The other guy left and I went back to get a battery charger I wanted for myself. As I climbed out, I saw Pop's car driving off. I looked down the alley the other way just as a police car turned in. *Shit,* I thought, and tossed the charger back inside. I turned to face the wall and acted like I'd been peeing there.

The cop drove up along side and said, "What you doing, Buddy?"

"Just taking a leak," I answered, turning around, trying to look innocent.

"Have to take the fan out to take a leak?"

"Hey, man, I don't know nothing about that."

"Yeah, sure," he said, getting out of the car. "Let's talk about this some more."

I got charged with the burglary, and from jail I called Bett and told her to go and get my cut from Pop. She later told me that Pop said, "There ain't no cut for him. You get caught, you're out."

When I went to court, my legal aid lawyer said, "This really isn't a big deal. You don't have any prior felonies, so we ought to be able to get you off with probation. If you tell the judge you have a drug problem he'll probably send you to a hospital instead of jail."

Maybe the lawyer didn't think it was a big deal, but I was scared to death. The idea that I could go to prison was terrifying. I'd heard stories … This was going to be the last time I ever got myself into something like this.

I followed his advice and ended up going to the Central State Mental Hospital in Petersburg, Virginia for thirty days of evaluation before I received a sentence; then I'd probably get two years of probation afterwards. The police took me to the hospital two days later on a cold, gray, rainy afternoon. As we drove by the low wall that surrounded the place, I saw several big three-story dark red brick buildings, all with heavy metal grates covering all the windows. Jagged black water stains dripped under each window, making the place look haunted, very depressing.

I was taken to a registration area that had a small counter for doing paperwork, and four or five chairs. A light-skinned guy was sitting there when I walked in; I sat down across from him while the nurse got some paperwork together for us. I put out my hand and said in a low voice, "Hey, man. Name's Billy Hairston."

"Hey, Bro," he said, shaking my hand. "Clarence."

"What you here for?" I asked in a low voice.

"Me?" he whispered, "I'm in for drugs. The judge sent me here. I just came so I could beat the rap."

"Me too!" I said. "I don't got no real problem. We can hang together, man. We can make it for thirty days." I raised my hand and gave him five.

After we'd finished the paperwork, a nurse took us through two locked doors to a dorm area with green linoleum floors and pale green walls. The patients' rooms surrounded a common area that held several metal tables with chairs and three or four heavy green vinyl couches, all ripped with the stuffing hanging out. One of the patients, an old man with a long gray beard, was sitting on one of them, staring into space. The nurse pointed out the showers and bathrooms as we walked by them, as well as two padded rooms that were really just cages. "These are just for the violent ones. You fellas want to stay outta there," she said. She showed us our rooms, each with a small dresser and single bed, told us to settle in, and she left.

When I went out to the common area, five or six patients were sitting around on chairs, some watching Truth or Consequences on a television mounted high on the wall; the rest just stared into space. Several wore faded pajamas, and the others were dressed in baggy clothing. One man paced up and down the side of the room, arguing with himself. I decided right off that I was going to stay away from those crazy people. Just looking at them made my stomach turn. *I sure as hell ain't like them*, I said to myself. I stood up straight and decided I'd be a macho bad guy, nothing at all like those nuts. *Nothing wrong with me*, I thought. *My drinking and drugging ain't a problem. I'm just here to stay out of jail.*

A nurse sat in a big overstuffed chair in an elevated glassed-in room off to one side where she could see the entire common area and the screened-in porch. She gave both Clarence and me papers to read that explained the rules, schedules and visiting hours. I sat down in the room with the other patients to read mine; Clarence headed out to the porch.

Sitting there, I became more aware of the constant underlying noise in that institution; it was like a loud hum, which I soon learned, never stopped. There were always people murmuring, crying, sobbing, screaming; and gates opening; doors clanging shut. I heard carts being pushed, silverware dropping, something being scraped across the floor, but couldn't tell where any of the sounds were coming from. It was odd, like something from science fiction. When we passed by the other wards on our way to the cafeteria, I learned those sounds were everywhere.

When I got into my narrow bed that night, I knew I wouldn't be able to sleep even though they'd given me a sedative. I had slept little since Vietnam, trying to avoid re-living the horrors in my head. The medication made me feel heavy and slow, groggy most of the time. After the second day, I hid the pills under my tongue at meds time and flushed them down the john first chance I got.

Two days later I was talking to one of the nurses at her desk when I saw Clarence go out to the porch. I followed him and sat down on one of the chairs that had been bolted to the wall and the floor. "Cold out here, ain't it?" I said.

He stood with his back to me, his fingers hooked into the blackened, soot-covered grid that enclosed the screens, staring out into the parking lot. He didn't seem to hear me.

"Man," I said. "I'll be glad when my thirty days are over." He didn't answer, so I got up and went back inside. Two orderlies, built like professional boxers dressed in white shirts and pants had arrived and were talking to the nurse.

About that time Clarence came back in and sat down on a couch away from everybody else. All of a sudden his face twisted up as if he was having a fit, he let out a scream and his body curled into a ball. The orderlies got up and headed toward him. It seemed to me that Clarence was trying to stretch out, then all of a sudden he jumped off the couch and flipped a heavy metal table over. Before the orderlies could reach him, Clarence tried to rip away two chairs that were bolted to the wall. He turned over everything he could put his hands on, jerked cushions off the sofas and sailed them through the air. Finally, the orderlies grabbed him.

With all three of them yelling, they dragged him down to one of the padded rooms.

The seven or eight other patients just sat there as if they hadn't even noticed what was going on. Those looking at the television kept watching; the ones staring into space didn't move. Clarence's desperate howls continued as I walked over to the nurse and said, "What's wrong with him? I came in with that guy."

"He's just having a reaction to coming off the drugs," she said, looking bored. "I can tell you, he's going to be here for quite a while."

"What are they doing to him?" I asked, listening to his terrified screams.

"They'll strip him and put him in a strait jacket. Give him some medication to calm him down, then take the jacket off. It sounds worse than it is."

I never saw Clarence again. And I didn't go looking for him, either. For the rest of my stay I was careful to avoid the other patients and follow all the rules. I met with the psychiatrist, did my group therapy, and sat near the nurse's station and talked to the staff.

The food was awful and I didn't eat in the cafeteria unless I was starving. Worse than the food was the fact that people were always starting fights, screaming and slinging macaroni and handfuls of jello at each other. Most of the time I got the nurses to buy me food on the outside, and I wrote Bett and my mom and asked them to send me something to eat.

During my second or third week, I ran out of supplies and was eating lunch, sitting by myself in the cafeteria, when one of the guys who had been standing in line walked over to the middle of the floor and started humming. He held his arms out like he was an airplane and rocked back and forth as he hummed louder and louder. "Hmmmmm, hmmmmm." After a few minutes, the others in the cafeteria started humming with him. With each hum, he rocked back and forth, further and further, until we could all see he was going to lose his balance. The orderlies, who were talking to each other, just watched with the rest of us till he fell backwards and slammed his head hard, into the concrete floor. The staff finished their conversation before two of them went over to him. After they realized that he wasn't conscious, one grabbed his arms, the other his feet, and they started walking out. The man's head fell back and to me he looked dead. After they were gone, someone else came in with a mop and wiped up the blood. I never saw that man again, either.

It was then that I decided I needed to actively put a plan together to get the hell out of there as soon as possible. I asked one of the nurses, "Say, how do they decide you're ready to leave here?"

"They'll ask you some questions," she said, stapling papers together.

"What questions?" I asked, leaning forward.

"Oh, like, they'll want to know if you smell or hear anything unusual."

"Hear something? Like what? Like voices?"

"Yeah," she said, "like voices. Maybe telling you to hurt yourself or somebody else. Or you might be smelling something weird. Like gasoline, or shit, or something like that."

"Okay. What else they want to know?"

She glanced sideways at me. "They'll ask about your appetite. And how you're sleeping at night."

"I'm in good shape then," I said to her. "I can pass that test and hardly even have to lie."

Every day we went outside for an hour to walk around the yard and get some fresh air. There was a pay phone not far from the building, which was the only phone patients could use, so there were usually four or five people in line. After I was given permission to have visitors, I went to the phone booth to call Bett. A man was already using it, but I was next in line so I figured I wouldn't have to wait long. I lit up a cigarette.

I'd just flicked the butt away when four young white kids came up, two guys and two girls. The most talkative guy was tall and blond with a bad case of acne, and wore one white tennis shoe and one black. The other boy was shorter and dark. The black-headed girl next to the tall kid looked like a tomboy; her socks were all down in her shoes and she wore dirty jeans and a flannel shirt. The other girl, dressed in black, was silent. They all wore baggy clothes that looked like they'd come out of a garbage can, and had long scraggly hair. The guys were unshaven and wore gloves with the fingers cut off. They looked to me like they were, uh, crazy.

"Hey, Brother," the blond guy said. "What's going on?" He reached out and attempted something like the Dap handshake but didn't know how to do it; we did our best and fumbled through. "You waitin' to use the phone?"

"That's right," I said.

"So, go on. Use the phone," he said. They all started beating on the phone booth and shouting at the man inside, "Hey, asshole, get the fuck outta there. The brother wants to use the phone." The guy looked up and then went back to talking.

I looked at the kids. "That's okay. I don't mind waiting," I said. "He'll be done soon."

"Naw, man. He's taking all day. Let's get him outta there!" said the shorter guy. They pushed the door open, grabbed him by the arm and pulled him out. As he ran off, the blond guy said, "Go on in, man. It's your turn now."

When I got in the booth, I picked up the dangling receiver and said hello but there was no answer. While I put my money in to make the call, the kids surrounded the phone booth and stood with their backs to me, daring anybody else to get in line. I managed to get Lee on the phone, and he said he'd bring Bett up, along with some groceries, on Sunday. As I stepped out of the booth I looked at the tall kid and said, "Thanks, man."

"Hey, where you going?" the tomboy said, putting her arm through mine. "You still got time. Come on with us."

I looked at my watch trying to think of some reason I couldn't go, but ended up saying, "Well, I got a few minutes. I guess so." After seeing what they'd done to the other man I wanted to be sure they thought I was their friend. I managed to unhook the tomboy from my arm and we started walking across the basketball court.

The taller boy said, "Bet you could play some basketball."

"Yeah," I said, "I can hit a basket or two."

He pointed over to an ancient brick building not too far from the unit I was in. "That's where we live," he said. "Right over there." We walked on in silence till we came to a wooded area where there was an old dirty mattress, a few broken chairs and a dresser with all the drawers missing. We could see the highway from there.

"Want something to drink? Got some Mad Dog, here," he said, pulling out a bottle from behind the dresser.

"No, thanks," I said. "Where'd you get that?"

"The liquor store. Hey, man. We go wherever we want. They ain't keeping us in here." After a minute, he pointed to the quiet girl and said, "Hey, that's my girlfriend, Shelly. You like her?"

"Yeah," I said looking at her filthy clothes, dirty face and tangled hair. "She looks real nice."

"Want to fuck her?" he asked.

"Oh, no, man," I said. "I couldn't do that man. I'm married."

"Come on. That don't matter," he said. "She don't care."

"No, man. Thanks, but that ain't right. I can't do that."

"What's the deal, asshole? She ain't good enough for you? Is that it?" He stood up and I thought he was coming for me.

"Oh, no, man. No way," I said. I knew I had to get out of this without insulting him. Or her. "Tell you the truth, man," I said, "it's the medication they got me on. You know how it is, man. I don't like to say it, but I just can't get it on right now."

"Oh," he said, sitting back down. "That's too bad, man. Next time, maybe."

"Yeah," I said, "next time." We talked a while longer and I looked at my watch. "Guess I got to go back," I said. "Don't want to be late and get in trouble. I might miss my visit on Sunday."

That was the last time I used that phone.

The following Sunday Lee drove up with Bett and met me down in the lobby. We couldn't leave the grounds, but we walked around together outside and had a little picnic. When it was almost time for them to leave, we went around to the back parking lot so Lee could show off his nice new Oldsmobile 225. When we got there, one side of the car was covered with mud. Just one side. The other side was fine. As we looked at it, the kids I'd met at the phone booth walked over.

"Hey, man," the blond kid said. "Looks like you need a car wash, dude."

I just shook my head.

"Only cost you seven bucks," he said. "Good deal."

I turned my back to him and whispered to Lee, "Sorry man, but those dudes are crazy. Just give them the seven dollars."

He handed them the money, and after they hosed off the car and left, he leaned over to me and said, laughing, "Now, Billy Junior, you just tell me who's the crazy ones! Them guys are acting awful smart to be crazy."

When my thirty days were up and I answered all the doctor's questions to his satisfaction, I was released. Bett and Lee picked me up, and this time he parked in the front parking lot. It felt so good to be free of that depressing place. It was as if there was no hope in there. None at all. As we drove away I promised myself that I'd never go anywhere like that again.

◆   ◆   ◆

Bett was still living with her parents, but when I got home she moved in with me and my mom, back into that cramped apartment. I was determined to find a job and stay out of trouble. I did my best but I thought constantly about the peace and comfort I'd felt when I was high on heroin or coke, and it wasn't long before I was using. Determined not to get hooked again, I tried limiting myself. I'd do heroin just once in the morning and once at night, thinking I could make do with gin and beer in between, but the more I tried to control it, the more I used. I'd force myself to think about the mental hospital because I knew I never wanted to go back there, but it didn't make any difference. I couldn't stop.

Unable to find work that could support my family and my drug habit, in desperation I decided it was time to make a career change. I moved from burglary to armed robbery. I held up small convenience stores and mom and pop establishments, always with an unloaded gun. I never even bought any bullets to put in the chamber. It was the easiest way to get fast cash for drugs, and I always went into it with the idea that if there was any problem, I'd just leave and go down the block to the next little store. I knew it was wrong, and I always felt guilty about what I was doing but that didn't stop me. I'd tell myself that after this one time I'd change my life, get a job and get off drugs, but as soon as my stomach started cramping in withdrawal or I started sweating because I needed a fix, I'd rob another store.

Usually, I'd just ask for money out of the register so I could get in and out quick; opening a safe took more time. I never got much, but I got out fast. My most notorious holdup was when I robbed a small convenience store where the cashier was a little old blond-headed lady who wore lots of makeup. She seemed friendly, moved slowly and spoke softly. When I was sure all the other customers had left, I walked up to the counter. She said, "My goodness, you're a tall one! How tall are you?"

I pulled my gun out and said, "Give me all your cash." She looked surprised and said, "Well, ain't got much in here. This ain't hardly gonna be worth your trouble."

I stepped around behind the counter as she handed me the few bills from the register, and I saw a moneybag on the floor. It was one of those sacks that people used back then to deposit money. It had a dollar sign on it, so I grabbed it too. It was so heavy it caught me by surprise and I almost dropped it. As I left the store, without thinking, I called back over my shoulder, "Thank you."

When I got home and opened the bag, I saw I'd stolen a bunch of pennies. Not what I had in mind, but it was better than nothing. It took me a couple of days to wrap them all, and when I finished I had two hundred dollars worth. One of the newspapers called me the "Piggy Bank Robber," but I didn't mind. The drug dealers didn't care if they were paid in pennies.

Backed Up Against the Wall

◆

1971–1972

I'd made myself a rule that when I robbed any store, I'd only go for the what was in the cash register. But when I was really desperate for a fix one afternoon, I decided to go for the money in the safe. It was about four or five o'clock, not the best time to rob a convenience store, but I was getting the shakes really bad and had to get some coke. I hung around looking at magazines till everybody left the place, then went up to the young Asian-looking cashier and pulled out my gun. "Gimme all your cash," I said.

Looking scared to death, the man opened the register, scooped out the bills and put them on the countertop. I pointed my gun at the safe and said, "Open that up! I want everything!" He turned around and was fumbling with the combination lock when I heard footsteps behind me. I looked toward the aisle and saw someone crouching, moving my way. I figured he must have a gun or some kind of weapon if he was coming after me, so I said, "Stop or I'll shoot!" Then I grabbed the money from the counter and ran out as fast as I could, zigzagging down the sidewalk, so I'd be hard to hit. The guy didn't yell or call out, but I heard the gunshots. I'd almost made it around the corner when I felt a tug and a push at my right shoulder.

A friend we called Dog was waiting for me in his car, so I jumped in and said, "Drive! Drive! Drive!" He shifted into gear and gunned the engine. I fell over in the front seat to hide, because to get away we had to pass the intersection where they'd been shooting at me. Dog looked over and said, "Man, you been hit."

I put my hand up to my shoulder and felt the warm, sticky blood. "Oh, shit," I said.

When we got home Bett and my mom weren't there, so we wrapped my arm in a towel to stop the bleeding and split the money, almost five hundred dollars. I gave Dog two hundred and he went to get some dope while I settled down on the sofa to have a beer. He was back in about twenty minutes and I was feeling okay by the time Bett got home.

When she saw the bloody towel, she was pissed. "What you done now, dumb ass?" she said. You know, your mama was right. You ain't no good at nothing but getting stoned. You're more goddamned trouble than you're worth."

To try to make things better, I gave her a hundred dollars, which she stuck in her pocket without a word, then put her hands on her hips and stared at me.

"I got shot," I said. "I need you to get the bullet out." She came over, removed the towel and gently touched my arm. "Try to move it a little," I said. "See if you can just squeeze it out." She squeezed hard and I gritted my teeth, then yelled, "OOWWW! Damn it!"

"I think it moved a little," Bett said. "But it ain't coming out."

"Try again," I said, wiping sweat from my brow. She squeezed my arm again, but when I yelled, she stopped.

"I can't do it. It won't move. I can't do it," she said.

"Then get a razor blade," I said, wiping my brow with the bloody towel, "and cut it out."

"You fucking crazy?" she said, backing away. "I ain't no doctor. I ain't cutting on you."

"Come on, Bett. Just make a little slit and pull it right out. It won't be hard."

"Then you do it," she said. "I'll get you the razor."

In the end, she went to the store and got some gauze and tape and bandaged my arm with the bullet still inside.

After Bett left to go to her sister's, Dog said, "Hey man, I heard there's a male nurse over at the projects who's as good as any doctor. Maybe he can fix you up as a favor."

"Worth a try," I said. "Give me another hit and let's go."

It took us an hour to find the guy in a dark, dirty apartment. As he examined my arm I could tell he didn't like the look of things. The first thing he said was, "How much money you got? No money, no help." I stood up and walked out. I needed my money for a fix.

When we got back, Bett was home. "So, how you gonna get that bullet out?" she asked.

"Can't do it around here," I said. "Gunshot wound. Any doctor would call the cops."

"Ain't you the genius," she said, her hands on her hips, just like her mother. "So how long you gonna lie around here on your ass, Mr. Big Shot? How you gonna feed your habit now? How you gonna pay the rent? How you gonna buy food? You sure as hell ain't gonna be getting a job with your arm like that."

"I got plans. Don't you worry, Bett. I got plans."

Two days later my money was gone and the only plan I'd come up with was to get out of town. I knew Clint and J.J. were both in Washington, D.C., where Clint was dealing drugs. I called him and asked if I could come to visit. He met me at the bus station and he was looking good. "Hey, Bro," he said, "I know about a hospital here where you can see a doc for free."

"They ain't gonna ask how I got a bullet in my arm?"

"Nah, man. It's cool."

"Let's go, then," I said as we got in his car. "I'm ready." When we'd gone about half a mile, a siren started wailing behind us.

"Shit!" Clint said. "I knew they was watching me. Goddamned motherfuckin' shit!" We pulled over and the officer, who had broad shoulders and an attitude, came up to the driver's window and said, "Well now, you fellas got a tail light burned out."

"I'm taking this man to the hospital," Clint said, pointing at me. "He got shot."

Broad Shoulders looked over at me and I lifted up my bandaged arm. "Okay then," he said. "Go on ahead. We'll follow you." He walked back to his car.

"Shit!" Clint said, pounding his fist on the steering wheel. "Goddamned cock-sucker. Listen, man, you tell them you got shot in a bar fight. At the Blue Moon. Some dude you never saw before."

"Right, man," I said. "Okay." I didn't like any of this, but figured I didn't have much choice.

When we drove into the Emergency Room parking area, the cops pulled up right beside us. As we walked to the door, Broad Shoulders said to me, "We need to take a report on this gunshot wound. I'll talk to you inside."

I looked at Clint and he shrugged his shoulders as we entered the hospital. I walked past ten or twelve other people who were sitting around waiting, and signed in at the desk. Then the officers waved at me to sit with them in some chairs off in a corner. They told Clint to move to another part of the room. The other cop pulled out a clipboard with a form on it and said, "All right, what happened here? Who shot you?"

"I was in this bar, The Blue Moon. I was just having a beer when this guy come in and started a fight with another guy."

"Big guy, was he?"

"Kinda' big, yeah." I said.

"What's he look like?"

"Big, like I said. Light-skinned."

"Hmm. Did he have any tattoos of a girl on his arm?"

"Yeah, I think he did," I said, screwing up my face like I was trying to remember. "Seems like maybe he did."

"Hear anybody call his name?"

"Naw, man. He just started yelling like he was crazy. Next thing I knew he pulled out a gun and started firing so I ran the other way as fast as I could. Almost got outside, too." The officers looked at each other and I knew I was in way over my head.

"Got some ID?" he asked. I handed him my driver's license and he said, "Listen here, I want to make a deal with you. We think we know this fella who shot you, and we want to get him, bad. Now, if you'll help us, I'll give you the benefit of the doubt, and we won't run an ID on you."

I didn't really believe him, but figured I'd better act like I did. "So, what do I have to do?"

"I want you to wear a wire. This fella you described is in that bar every night. He's a drug dealer strong arm and we can't get anything on him. We just want you to have a little conversation with him, get him to admit to shooting and hitting you by mistake."

Goddamnit, I thought. *No fucking way.* "I don't know, man," I said, looking down at the floor and shaking my head. "Sounds like a quick way to get myself killed."

Broad Shoulders stood up. "All right, man. Your choice. You sit right here while I go run an ID."

I knew he had me. "Okay," I said, and he sat back down. "All right. I'll do it."

"Good," he said, motioning to his partner. "We'll go get everything set up. Be right back."

As soon as they left the waiting room, Clint and I walked to the front of the hospital and kept on going. "They got my license number," Clint said, "and they're gonna be looking for me, so you ain't gonna be able to stay at my place."

"Right, man. Maybe J.J. would let me hang out there."

When I got a hold of J.J., he said I could stay with him and his sister for a few days, but I could tell he didn't like the idea. After all, they'd be harboring a fugitive with a bullet in his arm. I wasn't surprised when they asked me to leave early the next morning. I had nowhere to go but back home.

As I rode the bus back to Portsmouth, I tried to figure out a place I could stay. It couldn't be with my mom, because the law was after me. I still had the Pep

Boy's case pending, and the cop's snitches had probably told them I did the convenience store robbery. Bett had moved back in with her parents and I knew I couldn't stay there. And even if I could, the cops would go there looking for me. I'd have to ask friends.

As it turned out I kept moving around, staying two days here and three days there. When I had money or drugs it was easy to find a friend, but now that I was broke it was a different story. The police had long ago made a practice of stopping whenever they saw a few of us black men standing on a street corner, and a couple of times I'd managed to ease away when I saw them coming. But within two weeks, I got picked up. The officer, who looked familiar, walked up to me and said, "Hey, man, how was D.C.?"

"What? What you talking about?" I asked.

"Still got that bullet in your arm?" he said.

"Bullet? I don't know what you talking about, man,"

When he reached over and hit my shoulder, I yelled out in pain. He took me in for questioning and a nurse at the jail removed most of the bullet—when it rains I'm reminded that there's still a small piece there.

I couldn't make bail, so I stayed in the overcrowded jail that stank with the smell of unwashed bodies. Peeling yellow paint covered the walls. Every cellblock had ten cells, each one intended to hold one man. There were five cells along each side of a wide hall. All had metal bunks attached to the wall and each had a toilet. In the middle of the hallway was a table for meals, where we ate in shifts. A toilet and a shower were at the end of the hall and there was a television high on the wall that the inmates could see.

But at that time, the cellblock held about fifty men instead of the ten it was built to house, and most of us slept on the floor on one-inch green foam mattresses with a sheet and blanket, and if you were lucky, a pillow. Those who couldn't find a place in the cells slept in the hallway, some under the table.

I told them I was afraid I'd be going through withdrawal there, so for the first three days they put me on a different floor, in a cell with a real door, where I could be alone. Once a day the nurse checked my blood pressure, but that was their only concern. They gave me nothing to help with the absolutely indescribable hell of withdrawal: the shakes, paranoia, panic attacks, hot and cold flashes, unquenchable thirst, a lot of puking, and hallucinations.

When I got down to the cellblock on the fourth day, the other inmates helped some, bringing me food and drink, sharing their blankets for the cold flashes, talking to me, telling me I could make it through. Eight months later I went to court to face my charges.

Originally I'd been charged with eight armed robberies but only three of the people picked me out of the lineup. The police told me that the woman I'd stolen the pennies from said, "He was such a nice robber; he even said thank you. I really didn't want to tell on him."

I was scared to go to court but I did my best to act macho, like I was a tough guy. They were only prosecuting me on three of the armed robberies, plus the Pep Boys burglary, but I knew this was big time. The morning of the hearing I was hauled over to the courthouse with a van full of prisoners who all had court dates. I tried to look like I wasn't worried, like I had it all under control, but I knew I was in for it this time. I met my lawyer about five minutes before I was to appear before the judge.

He walked up to me and said, "Hairston. That you?"

"Sure is," I said.

"All right now," he said, looking at me and reaching his hand out to shake mine. "I'm Marcus Lowery, your lawyer. Haven't had a chance to read your file. What are the charges?"

"Three counts of armed robbery and one count of midnight burglary," I said.

"Hmm." He opened the file. "I assume you're guilty?"

"Yeah," I said.

He flipped through the pages, then said, "I recommend you take a plea bargain. It's gonna look stiff at first, but I'll go ahead and set a date to get the sentence reduced."

"Think that's the best I can do?"

"Looks that way now," he said. "If you stay outta trouble the first few months, there's a good chance we'll get a reduction."

"Okay," I said. "How much time will I get?"

"You're looking at twenty-six years. Eight for each armed robbery and two for the burglary."

I felt like somebody had hit me in the gut with a tire iron. I took a step back. "What the fuck? Twenty-six years?"

"And that's just because the detectives say you aren't the career criminal type. But we'll get it reduced. You'll end up with ten or less, I'd guess."

The courtroom door opened and a man in a black suit waved at us. "We're coming," Lowery called out, then he turned back to me. "When we go in, you sit down on the front row. Then when the bailiff calls you, I'll show you where to go. Don't say anything till I tell you. I'll do the talking and you only answer the judge if he asks you something. Which he won't."

"Yes, sir," I said, still stunned. "All right."

While I sat waiting, dreading what was coming, I looked at the judge, an old man with a red face who wore half-glasses down on the tip of his nose. He looked very imposing, but I couldn't decide whether he looked mean or not. When they called my name, Lowery pointed the way and I went up and stood next to him. But from that point on I just looked at the floor. The only time the judge spoke to me was to sentence me to twenty-six years.

I went back to the holding area, built for ten people but holding about forty. We had to wait there till everyone's court hearing was finished, which took about five hours. During that time the reality of what I had done to myself started sinking in. I felt like my life was over. It got harder and harder to keep up my macho image talking to the others, so I sat on the floor and leaned up against the wall and pretended I'd gone to sleep. What I really wanted to do was curl up in a ball and cry.

When we finally got back to the jail, I was put in a single cell in the cellblock all by myself, as was the custom for someone receiving a sentence like mine. I was finally separated from the others in the overcrowded block and the relief was overwhelming. I could quit pretending that I didn't care what was happening to me. I lay down on the bed, covered my head with a blanket and silently cried myself to sleep.

A few hours later I woke up to the sound of a woman's voice singing softly, "Come into my heart, into my heart, come into my heart, Lord Jesus." I opened my eyes and looked through the bars of my cell. There stood a short, plump, dark-skinned woman singing on the visitor's side of the bars, one of the religious missionaries who were allowed in to visit the inmates. All the other prisoners had moved away from her and gathered down at the television set. She was looking right at my cell. It was so comforting to me, like a quiet sign that I'd be all right.

The next day I went right back to my macho act.

I spent the first eight months of my sentence in processing before being sent to the State Prison in Richmond they called "The Wall." Then I'd be sent on to a Work Camp. Everybody talked about how horrible The Wall was, and I was relieved I'd only have to be there for a week. The most dangerous criminals were kept there and I'd heard it was like a dungeon. Rumor was that because the inmates had such long sentences, the feeling of hopelessness sucked the life right out of you. To survive in that place you had to have a reputation of being tough, and the thought of being transferred there filled me with dread.

When the day came, six other men and I, all in shackles, were transported to The Wall in a van. We were led down a long gray corridor through five locked metal gates; the one ahead of us wouldn't open until the one behind us clanged shut. When we'd gone through the last one, we entered an open area that was surrounded by cells. Men yelled at us, "Come over here, cocksucker! You gonna be my new bitch," and "You the nigger turned me in? I'm gonna kill you, motherfucker." They made comments about our asses and what they were going to do to us. One guy was already selling us for two packs of cigarettes.

The guards were rough and harsh and they shouted orders that they expected to be obeyed immediately. It was clear that their goal was to humiliate us and show us they were in control while we were powerless. They got their message across.

On my third day in the Admissions Unit a bunch of us new arrivals, all in shackles, were lined up in a hallway getting ready to go to the cafeteria for lunch. The other prisoners were milling around in the common area, talking and playing cards. All of a sudden an inmate who was small but looked like a pro boxer, started shouting at one of the guys in our line, raced over with a knife and slammed him against the wall. "I told you I'd kill you, you bitch!" he yelled. "You ain't getting away this time, you cocksucker!"

Since we were all shackled, the victim couldn't raise his arms to defend himself and none of us could help him. The boxer stabbed him repeatedly in the chest and ran off. The man fell to the floor, covered with blood. Immediately, there was a hush in the hall. Then all hell broke loose; alarms clanged, the loudspeakers blared, "Lockdown, lockdown!" Doors and gates slammed shut, sounding like thunder. Nightsticks hit the cages. Men pushed each other, fell down, and ran to get the fuck out of there.

Serious Time

♦

1972–1973

Brick and concrete prisons were reserved for those who had ten years or more to serve, and since I'd appealed my sentence, I was transferred from The Wall to a less secure site, Work Camp 3, which was located in a farming area. We lived in a long, ancient wooden building with a flat tin roof. We slept in a room that could pass for a dormitory, bunk beds lined up in long rows. It was so shabby that when we cleaned up, we just swept the dirt through the cracks in the floor.

New inmates lived in the "gun side" of the building, where everyone was under armed guard. The lights were on twenty-four hours a day, which kept me on constant alert. Prisoners were never alone, were never out of sight of the guards or other prisoners; we were always exposed. We had to ask permission for everything. If I was lying on a bed and wanted to pass a book to my buddy on the upper bunk, I had to call over to the guard, "Hey, Boss. Passing up a book," and he'd nod. We had absolutely no rights. We had to stay on the gun side till we'd served a month for each year of our sentences, that is, nine months for a nine-year stretch. Then, the prisoners who kept themselves out of trouble were eligible to move to the "trustee side," where there were more privileges. Eventually, with good behavior, we'd be eligible for furloughs, where we could go home with our families for a few days at a time.

When I first got there, they still used balls and chains. When the shackles came off at night, the guards manacled us to the beds. The chains reached from one bed to the next, so that when one man turned over in his sleep, it pulled on the other men's ankles. It was really hard to get comfortable. To go to the bathroom, I had to raise my hand and a guard would unlock me from the chain. When I returned, he chained me back up.

After I'd been there two weeks the law was changed so that they couldn't chain us up at night anymore, but we still had to wear shackles when we were transported anywhere. They weren't tight, but they were heavy and cumbersome and scraped our ankles raw.

A number of the men at Camp 3 were violent and seemed to have no conscience, no remorse about anything they had done. They were the hardened criminals, the violent abusers and strong-arm men. They were said to be "of criminal mind" and were to be avoided at all cost.

But many of the others were there because of their addictions. They weren't experienced criminals and didn't know how to break the law without getting caught. They robbed and stole for drug money. During their time in the joint they often became angrier and more violent than they'd ever been on the streets.

There were two distinct sets of rules in prison. One was enforced by the prison guards and the other set down by the prisoners themselves. Since these two systems were often in opposition to each other, day-to-day life could be very precarious, like walking through broken glass. When the establishment rules were disobeyed, the penalty could mean additional time. When the inmates' rules were disobeyed, the penalty could be death. To inmates, unwritten laws included where to sit at dining room tables, who had first choice at anything and everything, how to participate in certain activities and games, who was on which team, and who could and could not be approached. Every inmate had to learn to walk a very narrow line.

Within the prison establishment itself, there was always the danger of getting on the bad side of one of the guards. There were liaisons between the inmates and the guards, and then there were friendships among the guards themselves. If one of the guards was angry with an inmate, other guards would go after that prisoner. The same was true when an inmate in one group got angry with an inmate in another group.

We worked in road gangs, cleaning out the ditches on large farms in the area and building interstate roads. It was hot, backbreaking labor, but I adjusted better than many because I'd learned how to deal with the heat in Vietnam. I knew to keep my shirt on no matter how hot it got and to take little sips of water instead of gulping it down and then getting sick. What was harder for me than working in the heat, was the fact that the ditches often had snakes in and around them. The thought of stepping on a snake still makes me break out in a sweat.

Even in prison, I remembered what my Uncle James and my high school basketball coach, Coach Sticky, taught me about putting forth my best effort, and I did that, whether I was digging ditches or cutting down trees or cooking in the prison kitchen. I never had a problem with working, I just had a problem living.

I couldn't get comfortable in my own skin. The only thing that ever helped was getting high.

Three months after I got there, as the lawyer promised, we went back to court on my appeal. Because it was my first prison sentence, and in part because of good behavior, it was determined that I was "not of criminal intent." The judge agreed to run the three eight-year sentences concurrently, and reduce the two-year sentence to one. That cut my time to nine years. Back then, for each year you only had to serve three months, so I figured I'd have to put in a total of about three and one-half years.

I'd turned eighteen in Vietnam and I turned twenty-one in a Virginia State Prison. I worked hard to be friendly but not too friendly, to blend in but not actually be a part of any group. I'd first learned that skill in elementary school. I never felt like I fit in, so I moved around the playground from one bunch of kids to another, not really joining any of them. That's exactly what I did in prison and it helped me to survive.

Prison is a scary place and being challenged by the other inmates is pretty much standard procedure. At each facility I got in fights, even after doing my best to avoid them, but after I proved myself they left me alone. Even though I wasn't heavy, being one of the tallest men there turned out to be more of a problem than an asset, because it was seen as a real accomplishment to get the best of one of the bigger inmates. I had to be careful about who I talked to, what I said, what area I was in, and who I was seen with. A glance in the wrong direction at the wrong time could get me beaten up. A comment in the wrong place or to the wrong prisoner or guard could get me killed.

Being kind and helping others were considered signs of weakness. Penitentiary life was hard, degrading, and very dangerous. I was afraid of the other prisoners, all seventy-six of them. I did my best to sleep with one eye open, which wasn't really much different from what I'd been doing since I got back from Vietnam.

Men who broke the prison regulations were considered role models by the other inmates; those who followed all the rules were cowards. It was weak to take responsibility for something; it was always somebody else's fault. If somebody was "weak enough" to be caught praying, he'd get comments like, "What makes you think God helps people like us? Now you want to get religion. God helps those who help themselves."

The smartest men were the ones who figured out how to stay within the rules and get all of those privileges, yet still find ways to get around the regulations so they wouldn't be considered weak. For example, anybody coming back from visiting home on a furlough had the best opportunity to bring drugs in, and everybody wanted them to bring something back. So, the month before an inmate was scheduled to leave, he was very popular.

The dumb ones refused to bring back anything but their own drugs, which they planned to sell. Not only was their stuff taken away by the other prisoners, they were often beaten or even killed. The smartest men agreed to bring back everybody's stuff along with their own. They'd distribute the drugs to the other men, wait till they'd all been sold, and then, when they could charge more, sell their own stuff.

While I was incarcerated I started attending Alcoholics Anonymous (AA) meetings for the first time. Mostly I went for the coffee and donuts. I was fascinated with the people who spoke in the meetings, getting little bits and pieces of knowledge that sometimes hit a chord. I knew I was an addict but I didn't really believe that I was an alcoholic. In spite of that, I thought I could learn a little bit from AA's Twelve Steps and figure out a program I could work on my own. They said that to work the steps you had to admit that you were powerless over drugs or alcohol, make a decision to change your life, and accept responsibility for your actions. All of them: present, past, and future. All I wanted to do was to stop drinking and using; I didn't need to worry about all that other stuff.

Because it was a good way to keep to myself out of trouble, I started reading again at Work Camp 3. It was a great way to escape from the reality of my life. I didn't just read the books, I lived the books. I was Ahab looking for Moby Dick, Sinbad sailing the Seven Seas, I was Hannibal—General of Armies, I was Napoleon the Conqueror. I learned to solve murder mysteries. I read romance novels and imagined I had a beautiful woman and a big estate, that I was rich and famous. From books I picked up ideas on a wide range of topics, from etiquette to medical terminology. Books and TV were my learning tools and helped me learn other ways to live, from the proper way to hold a fork, to how to speak with passion.

My best friend there was Chin Daddy, a huge bald man with a funkadelic braided goatee that he often laced with beads. He was from Chesapeake, which was close to Portsmouth, so we hung out together. He was a jovial sort, always laughing, and was one of the few men I could play checkers with who wouldn't flip the table over if I beat him.

Because he was new and only doing a two-year bit, the others gave him a hard time; the toughest months in prison are the first few and the last few. When an inmate is new, the others constantly test him to see how much he can take. When his time is about up and he wants to be careful not to screw up his release, the others know he won't make waves if they push him to his limit.

◆   ◆   ◆

One hot August morning the guards shackled Chin Daddy and me and three others for a work detail and took us out to a huge dump truck that held a big plywood box with some air holes cut in it. They lined us up, shoved us inside the box and locked it with a big padlock. The heat was awful. An armed guard sat in a chair next to the box with his rifle over his knees. We drove way out in the country, in the middle of nowhere and stopped by a weedy irrigation ditch in back of a cornfield. They unshackled us, gave us each a shovel, and led us to a ditch that was about twenty feet wide and filled with dark brown water that smelled like something huge had died in it.

One of the guards picked up a flat rock and said, "Hey, look at this, boys." He skipped it across the water and instantly the ditch was alive with snakes. There must have been a hundred of them in the weeds and grass. My heart started pounding and my skin crawled.

"Go on now," the guard said. "Get your asses down there and start digging. We got to get this cleared out by the end of the day."

"Hey, Boss Man," I said, looking over at him as I leaned on my shovel. "I ain't going in there with no snakes. Never bucked before, but today Boss, I'm bucking. I ain't going in that ditch." The guard pumped a round into his shotgun. I threw down my shovel, scared but trying not to show it.

"It's not that bad," Chin Daddy said. "You just make lots of noise and them snakes go the other way. They're scared of you."

The truck driver came up and got in my face. "What are you," he asked, "some kind of pussy? A city boy?"

"You call me whatever you want," I said, backing up. "I ain't going in there." One by one the other men decided they weren't going in either, so we ended up returning to the prison. The guards were really pissed.

I spent five days in solitary confinement, naked, in a hot, gray, windowless cell that had one weak light bulb in a ceiling that was so high it couldn't be reached without a ladder. The cell itself was four feet by four feet so I couldn't even sit down and stretch my legs out in front of me. There was a blanket to sleep on and a hole in the concrete floor to use as a toilet. One of the trustees delivered a tray of food twice a day; for breakfast I had bread and water, for dinner a bologna sandwich and a glass of milk. I was lucky though, because Chin Daddy paid the trustee to sneak me in a few candy bars.

Being in solitary was humiliating. That's the whole purpose of it. When they took all my clothes away, they took away any shred of dignity or self-respect I might have had left. The days and nights were endless and the boredom was awful. I'd think about one of the books I'd read, and escape to another place like I'd done years before when my mom locked me the closet. I hated being in that cell, but I never regretted my decision to refuse to go into that ditch. Not even when I felt the most hopeless.

When I got out I asked Chin Daddy, "What ever happened at that ditch? You guys ever have to go in with them snakes?"

"Naw," he said, laughing and slapping me on the back. "We never heard nothing else about it. And we didn't get no solitary, neither. They said you was the ringleader and the rest of us was just following you."

Not long after that, Chin Daddy was transferred to work release and I became an institutional cook, which gave me extra privileges and new skills that, they said, I could use to find work when I got out. Since I had access to food and other special things the men wanted, I felt safer, like I had more control over my life. So long as I got others what they asked for, they left me alone. And I even made a profit at the same time. I sold fruit and sugar to other prisoners who'd make up a mash and take it out in a field to ferment before they sold it or drank it. Mostly the guards didn't mind. Some even drank with us.

◆   ◆   ◆

The guards were supposed to eat the same prison food we ate, but if I fixed them hamburgers or steaks, they'd look the other way while I cooked up extra burgers to take back to the cellblock to sell. In many ways the guards were much like us prisoners. They lived on the prison grounds while they were on duty and worked three weeks on and one week off.

The inmates' principles were based entirely on how they could use the other men or what they could take from them. There was a mafia of sorts within the walls. It was all about intimidation. If someone lent me a dollar bill, which was technically considered contraband in prison, I had to repay him with two. Everything a prisoner or guard gave anybody had a price. Some inmates laid out their "territory" and if anyone so much as walked across it, he could lose his life.

Because drugs were everywhere, I was able to make some money by selling weed. I couldn't bring anything in when I came back from a furlough, but I'd get Bett to bring me some; she could buy an ounce of pot for twenty dollars and I could sell it for a hundred and twenty-five. She'd hide a bag of dope near a mile marker down the road from the prison gate and one of the trustees responsible for keeping that part of the yard clean would pick it up for me. For a small cut.

For one joint, I could get five packs of cigarettes, or a dollar, cash. If somebody wanted a cigarette and didn't have the money, I'd put it "on the book," and when he paid me back he'd have to give me three. When men didn't repay me, I had to decide which ones it was safe to approach. If I reminded the wrong man that he still owed me, or mentioned it to somebody at the wrong time, my life could be in danger. At the same time, if I kept giving cigarettes away, I'd be considered weak and could be targeted by the others. It was a fine line to walk.

I paid close attention to the men who were always in fights with those tough guys, and the reasons for the conflicts. Then I was careful not to get in those kinds of situations with them. Just talking to them could give somebody the idea that I was on their side. By being very careful and studying the behaviors of the other men, I usually managed to stay out of harm's way.

◆   ◆   ◆

One night six or seven of us were watching *Soul Train* on TV when a new guy, a fat, pale, mean-looking redneck stood up, reached high on the wall where the TV was mounted, and switched the channel to *Hee Haw*.

"Hey," yelled Riff, one of the tough black guys. "What the fuck you doing? Put that back!"

"I'm watching *Hee Haw*," the redneck said, narrowing his eyes at the group, daring us to say anything. Then he sat down in one of the chairs right in front of the TV.

"The fuck you are," Riff said, standing up. He changed the station back to *Soul Train,* then turned to the redneck and said, "Don't fuck with that set."

The redneck stood and changed the channel again, then sat back down.

We all saw the rage on Riff's face as he slowly got up and walked to his bunk. Everybody who was sitting near the redneck immediately got up and left, and I followed them, looking back over my shoulder. When Riff returned, he walked up behind the new guy, stabbed him three times in the neck and ran off. The few men still there scattered and by the time the redneck hit the floor, he was the only one in the area. *Hee Haw* was still blaring away.

When the guards found him lying there dead, they hauled his body away. They asked who had been around when it happened, but only got answers like, "Man, I was lying on my bunk, looking the other way. I didn't see nothing," or "I was writing a letter." To say anything different would have been a death sentence.

We walked on eggshells for three days, till somebody caved in and told them it was Riff, and they took him away. During the years I was incarcerated after that, I never once tried to change the TV channel.

◆   ◆   ◆

I didn't watch as much TV after the *Hee Haw* incident. Instead, a bunch of us sat around in the evenings, playing cards and talking, and I got myself a good education in how to be a professional criminal. Living with a bunch of them, it was easy to pick up new ways to make a living on the outside.

Aunt Lena wrote to me a few times, telling me to trust in God and everything would be all right. And although they never wrote, my mom and Bett always visited me in prison. We'd sit at picnic tables and I'd listen to Bett tell me how hard it was out there, and about all her troubles. Her complaining reminded me of the letters she'd written to me when I was in Vietnam, all full of bad news. My mom never said much, but she usually left me a few dollars, not enough to buy anything, but her intention was good.

One Sunday when they came to visit me, Bett was in a great mood. As usual, we were sitting at a picnic table outside in the yard with all the other families. My mom was at a different table, but nearby. Bett looked at me with her big, dark eyes and said, "I got some great news, baby. You won't believe it!"

"What's that? I asked.

"Remember that last furlough you were on? You're gonna be a daddy," she said, hugging me. "I'm pregnant."

Immediately, I was bursting with pride. "Hey, Baby, that's great!" I said, getting up and hugging her. I looked over at my mom and smiled, but she just looked back with a blank face.

Later, after I'd told all my buddies the news, I started to wonder if the kid was really mine, because I didn't think we'd been together at the right time. Bett swore it was my baby, that she'd gotten pregnant when I was at home and I wanted to believe her. I was pretty sure she was lying, but I didn't make a big deal out of it. It was easier to pretend.

For the last four or five months of my sentence I was transferred to Camp 22 in Chesapeake, where we were on work release with only a couple of guards supervising us. Then I was closer to Portsmouth—they'd just started a new program where they tried to move inmates nearer to home so that when they got out they might be able to keep the same jobs. Five other men and I were assigned to the Lone Star Cement Foundry that made huge columns for highway overpasses.

We were taken there by bus on our first day, and the supervisor assigned us to different teams. When my team walked out to meet our foreman, I was surprised to see it was Chin Daddy. We both smiled and shook hands but acted like we didn't know each other. On the lunch break he told me to follow him to the parking lot.

We stood beside his blue Ford Mustang and talked a few minutes, then he reached in his pocket and handed me the car keys. "Go have a little fun," he said, "but be back by 3:30." I headed to the nearest bar and had myself a few.

Until I finished my bit, he signed me out on the weekends for extra jobs. Sometimes I worked and a few times I went home "on furlough" and partied with him and Bett.

Lost

◆

1973–1980

When I was released, Bett came to pick me up with our new baby girl who she affectionately called Puff. "This time," I said to Bett, "I'm gonna get a real job and stay clean. I got three years parole and I've had enough of this shit. I'm through with drugs."

Bett had managed to get a small garage apartment, which was good, but I had no decent clothes to wear job-hunting, and no car. I borrowed money to buy a shirt and pants, and found rides or took the bus to apply for jobs. I knew when I found work I'd need to have a way to get there, and much of the work was at construction sites a far distance away. But that was a problem for later.

When I filled out my first application, I came face to face with a major problem. One of the questions was, "Have you ever been convicted of a felony?" At first, I answered honestly, which I quickly saw kept me from ever getting an interview. Then I started lying, and a few times even got hired, then fired within a couple of weeks when they found out about my criminal record.

Discouraged, I started going to interviews with an attitude, thinking over and over that they wouldn't hire me, and that it didn't matter since they were all minimum wage jobs anyhow I wouldn't be earning enough to support us. Although that way of thinking may have kept me from getting hired, the repeated rejections made me more and more defensive, and my inability to get any work set off a terrible depression.

At my lowest points I thought I'd be better off incarcerated, where I had rules and regulations to follow and there was some sort of organization to my daily life. In some ways I thought it had been easier in Vietnam.

When I first got out of prison I didn't use hard drugs, but I'd never intended to stop drinking. I just wanted to stay out of trouble and it seemed to me that the drugs were what caused my problems. I went sporadically to AA and Narcotics Anonymous (NA) meetings, even raised my hand and talked some. But at home after the meetings I drank wine while I listened to audiotapes on how I could stay sober, live one day at a time, and change my life. I thought a lot about which parts of the twelve step programs I could fit into my life, but I didn't think much about how I could change my life to fit into them.

I was back using heroin and cocaine when I got hired by the Hare Krishnas, unloading their banana boats four or five months later. To get hired, you stood at one of the gates each morning and they selected people who could work for as many hours as they wanted. I always worked hard and did a good job; once I worked there three days and nights straight because I was afraid I wouldn't get picked again.

One afternoon my supervisor called in sick, as he did often, and one of the owners asked me to take over. I was excited to have a chance to show what I could do. That same night I was helping stack some boxes when I heard a scream from over at the conveyor belt, "Heeeelllp, help me!!" I looked up to see other workers gathering around a woman who was leaning over the belt. They were yelling, "Where's the shut off? We can't find the shut off!" I raced over to the woman who was still screaming hysterically. She was wearing a blouse with a long cord at the neck that had gotten caught in the conveyor belt.

The workers kept yelling as they tried to pull her away, but the harder they tugged, the tighter the cord was pulled. It looked like she might be choked to death. I grabbed a box cutter, pushed my way up to her, and cut the cords. Even after she was safe, she kept screaming and crying, "Oh, my God, I could have died! Oh mother of Jesus! Oh, my God!" The other workers gathered around and we all comforted her. Right away we located the Emergency Stop button and made sure everybody knew where it was. Then I reminded the workers, "This is why you should wear the recommended kinds of clothing, nothing hanging loose, and no strings."

When the owners heard what I'd done, they invited me to the next supervisor's meeting. I dressed real nice that day and was surprised and very proud of myself when they gave me my boss's job. I liked the responsibility and started putting in ninety to a hundred hours a week. Not long after that the FDA Inspectors came, and when the line I supervised hit their specifications right on the head, I was promoted to Wharf Foreman. At last, I was having some success. My hard work was paying off and because I was using drugs, I could work all day and all night. It felt great to be able to support my family.

◆   ◆   ◆

Although work was going okay, things weren't good at home. I'd stopped going to AA and NA and was back into cocaine and heroin. I kept telling myself that I could stop before I got hooked. But I couldn't. When I got a craving, I'd try to have sex to get my mind off the drugs, but that didn't help for long. Besides, when I was on coke and smack I could keep the sex going forever—I felt really macho.

I tried to control my drinking by giving Bett all my money. On Fridays she'd buy me a case of beer, a half-gallon of gin, and a gallon of wine, then keep the rest of the money. When that wasn't enough for me to make it through the weekend, I'd nag her till she'd finally give in and go buy more.

When I could see that giving her money wasn't going to help, I tried giving it to my mom instead, which made it a lot harder to get it back. But in the end, she gave into my ranting and raving, too.

Sometimes I'd manage to get some hard stuff, and after using I'd be so ashamed and disgusted with myself that I'd throw my drug paraphernalia out of the car as I passed a vacant lot. That way I figured I'd never be able to find it again. Almost always, within hours I was out there in the dark with a flashlight or a cigarette lighter, looking for my stuff.

Bett and I argued all the time. Most nights she left Puff with her sister, got dressed up and went out alone. She always said I could come along, but only because she knew I wouldn't. I still couldn't tolerate being in crowded places. Sitting home by myself, I'd think about how she was cheating on me and work myself into a rage. Then I'd take another shot of heroin or smoke another joint and drink, just to calm myself down. Because she was my wife, I thought Bett should be more understanding and considerate of my problems, but instead she just did what she wanted to do.

Eventually, my drug use caused me to lose the Wharf Foreman job at the docks. I was home alone one night when Bett came in found me wasted again. She yelled, "You ain't nothing but a drug addict! Choose me or the drugs. You can't have both!"

"I know, I know," I said for the hundredth time. "Bett, I hate being like this. I hate myself. I want to stop." That was the truth, but I lied when I said, "I was clean for almost three weeks this last time."

"Don't matter," she said. "You don't never stay clean."

"But I want to. I try. Honest to God, Baby. I do my best."

"And this here is your best? Well, it ain't good enough."

I put my head in my hands. "What can I do? What would work?" I went round and round in my head, thinking, *Fuck her.*

No, she's right; I'm no good.

No, no. I got to be strong. I need treatment, that's all.

Why am I so weak? I'd be better off dead.

The next morning Bett suggested, "Why don't you go someplace else? Get out of here, away from all your druggie friends?"

I looked up at her. I hadn't thought of that. "That's a good idea. Maybe it would work. That's one thing I ain't tried." Somewhere Bett found me a thousand dollars for the trip; I bought a bus ticket to California and figured that the three days it would take me to get there would get me detoxed. After that, I'd have the will power to stop for good and could start my life over. The ride was terrible; I was sick and shaking all over, but I didn't use. When I got off the bus in Los Angeles I was sick. I felt like shit and I hadn't decided what I was going to do once I got there. I sat down on a bench and was trying to come up with a plan when a woman walked up to me.

"Tree?" she said. "Tree, is that you?"

I looked up into the face of Marlene, who had been in some of the NA meetings in Portsmouth. She had an apartment full of dope and lots of contacts, and I had a pocket full of money. That was the end of getting sober. After two weeks with her, I called Bett for bus money to get back home. On the ride back I found a guy who had a sack of reefer and some vodka, so I made it home without the shakes.

I honestly wanted to do better, to get myself straightened out. My life was built on good intentions, but I never followed through. That quiet voice inside my head kept telling me that the only way to change was to get clean but I couldn't do it. I begged God to make me a stronger man, to give me will power, to help me stop. Then I'd tell myself, *Just a little weed to take the edge off. This time I'll be able to control myself.*

I thought about drugs constantly, determined not to let them run my life. But when I got any money together at all, some switch went off in my brain and I had no control over my actions. The money always went for drugs. I couldn't hold down a job. It looked like the only job I could stick with was selling drugs.

◆   ◆   ◆

I was looking in the bedroom dresser drawer for some matches one day when I found a letter Bett had written but never mailed to Blow, a guy she knew from high school. "You know how much I love you," it said. "I hope some day we'll be able to raise our baby girl together." Although I'd long suspected that Puff wasn't my child, when the letter confirmed it I went into a tailspin. I finally found Bett at her parents' house that night. I grabbed her by the arm and took her outside, then held up the letter and shouted, "What the fuck is this?"

"What's that? How the hell would I know?" she yelled back.

"'Cause you wrote it. It's a letter."

"Yeah? What letter?"

"One you wrote to Blow."

She looked confused for a second, then tried to grab it from my hand. "Lemme see that," she said as I pulled it back from her.

"What you write him about Puff?" I yelled.

"You got no right to go into my shit!"

"I got no right? I got no right? You saying here Puff ain't my kid! You out fucking anybody and everybody. You been lying to me all this time. You knew …"

"And why not? You ain't nothing but a goddamned druggie."

I crushed the letter and threw it at her, then stalked off and went to get high. She went back inside. The next day I moved back in with my mom and Ivy, but I argued as much with them as I had with Bett. Life was nothing but one battle after the next. It didn't matter where I was living. I hated my family and I hated myself. I decided I'd had enough. Suicide was the only solution. *That'll show them,* I thought.

I found my mother's Valium and took the whole bottle, put a suicide note on my bed, and lay down to die. As I got drowsy, I thought to myself, *They'll be sorry. Look what they drove me to. They'll be better off without me.*

Later I learned that Ivy had come to my room to borrow some money, and when she found the note and couldn't wake me up, she called my mom. Together, they took me to the hospital, where once again, the doctors pumped my stomach and sent me home.

Within a few days I moved back in with Bett and started selling weed again. Bett said the letter to Blow was a lie, that she was mad at me and that's why she'd written it. She had left it in the drawer for me to find back then, and had forgotten about it. She'd never intended to mail it.

◆   ◆   ◆

I ended up opening my own bootlegging and drug house in the projects. I sold reefer, beer, liquor, wine, and drugs and had two other guys working for me in their apartments. But the police were on to us before long. I was pretty good at staying ahead of the law; I paid some of the neighbors to hide drugs in their apartments so I wouldn't get caught with them in my place. But I knew the cops were determined to nail me; within two months they caught me dealing and I went back to jail.

By the time I got out on bond, Bett had been evicted because the rent hadn't been paid. I ended up going back to my mother's and Bett went off with one of her boyfriends. Eventually I was sentenced to another six years in prison.

◆   ◆   ◆

Going to prison the second time was easier because I knew what to expect. This time I went to Camp 27, right outside of Richmond. Everybody, the guards and the prisoners, were all on drugs. People even came from outside to buy dope there. It was a very scary place; it was nothing to get raped, beaten up or even killed. The guards didn't break up fights or do anything to help the inmates, because they were too busy protecting themselves. I hardly slept during my time there.

As before, I didn't dare try to sneak anything in when I came back from furlough but when Bett visited she brought drugs for me to sell. She'd stash the stuff in the women's bathroom in the visiting area, up high in a little nook between the wall and the ceiling. I had a deal with the trustee who cleaned those bathrooms, and he'd pick the stuff up that night and give it to me. By the time I got out of there three years later, I'd saved enough money to buy a car.

When I was released, once again determined to stay straight, Bett came and picked me up. It felt so good to walk out those doors with her, back into the world again. I'd paid my debt to society and was a free man. I had my whole future ahead of me. This time I was determined to do it right. This time I'd make it.

As we walked to the car, Bett looked up at me and said, "Think I look different?"

I looked down at her. "Yeah, Baby. Looks like you picking up some weight."

She smiled and said, "You know something? Every time you come home on furlough, I get pregnant."

I stopped walking. "You're what?"

She patted her stomach. "That's right, baby. You're gonna be a daddy again. Now you got two babies."

I wanted to believe her. I really wanted to believe it was mine, but I didn't trust her. "Hmm," I said. "This is mine? You sure?"

"Sure, I'm sure," she said, looking hurt as she put her arm around me. "'Course you're the daddy. You know when you come home, that sperm is strong." She patted the front of my pants. "You sure know how to work it, Baby."

That was all I needed. I'd been incarcerated so long it didn't take much to get me excited. I thought for a minute. "But the only furlough I had was just a couple of months ago," I said.

"I know, baby. It's something, ain't it?"

I couldn't face fighting with her again. Besides, I was so horny I would have accepted anything she said. "You wearing any underwear?" I asked.

"No," she said, as she grabbed my hand, "I sure ain't, Honey. She smiled and hugged me.

In the back of my mind I knew she was lying about the baby, but I just let it be.

When we got to the car, it felt great to slide in behind the wheel and take off down the highway. It was so good to be out of that fucking prison.

"Guess where I'm living now," Bett said. I looked over at her. "Got me a nice house."

"What you mean?"

"There's this guy, Earl Davis. I been working with him. Met him at your mom's house. He was renting a room there."

"You never said nothing about him. What you talking about?"

"I been putting him with some of your contacts."

"Hooking him up with my dealers? You crazy?"

"Just listen to me, Billy. Now that you're out, you can take over. With his money and your connections you're gonna do fine. And, I got a house and I got you a job too, managing a corner store."

"You got it all figured out, don't you?" I said, my anger rising. "How you get into all this?"

"I just started selling a little weed on the side with Earl," she said. "One thing and then another. I been doing pretty good, too. Where you think I got that weed I brought you?"

I was angry, now. "You got no business dealing." Staring straight ahead, I gripped the steering wheel. The blessed feeling of freedom was gone.

◆   ◆   ◆

Home again and selling reefer, I met a white dude who wanted to get into the drug business. I started managing one of his convenience stores and within a fairly short time I was managing all eight he had in the area.

I was living with Bett, but Earl was in charge of the drug business. He came and went as he pleased, and that included sleeping with Bett whenever he felt like it. When Earl was around I slept on the couch and they slept in the bed. When Earl wasn't there, Bett would have sex with me but we had to be careful not to let him know. Since I had nowhere else to go, I went along with it.

I still find it hard to believe I lived like that. In many ways I felt like I hadn't really gotten out of prison. I was just in a different kind of prison. I thought over and over, *Why did I ever think things would get better?*

I knew right from wrong. I had values and morals, but for some reason I was incapable of applying them in my life. I cannot begin to describe how humiliating it was to live that way. I felt lower than I'd ever felt. Less than dirt. I was ashamed of myself, knowing what my father would say if he could see me. He was already embarrassed to have me for a son.

I went to AA and NA meetings and tried to figure out how to stay clean, but I was still smoking pot and drinking. Old timers at the meetings told me to get completely away from alcohol and drugs. They said anything I put before my recovery I stood to lose. I didn't understand the meaning of that statement till years later.

I was able to stay off the hard stuff for a couple of months, till I had to have two wisdom teeth pulled. The dentist gave me some pain medication and I was off and running. I prayed, I begged God to take this obsession from me. I hated myself, was disgusted that I wasn't stronger.

Eventually the convenience stores I'd been managing were all shut down because of building code violations and I was out of work again. Desperate to earn money, I started taking clothing orders from people and boosting. I'd steal whatever they wanted and they'd pay me half the price of the original item, but that didn't make enough money. Finally, I went back to selling the hard stuff.

About that time, Earl moved in with his girlfriend Lorretta, but we were partners and we continued to sell drugs together. I was living with Bett, but Earl came and went as he pleased and that included sleeping with Bett whenever he felt like it. I still find it hard to believe I lived like that. When Earl was around, I slept on the couch and they slept in the bed. When Earl wasn't there, Bett would have sex with me but we had to be careful not to let him know.

Earl was taking over the drug business and paying our bills. He had complete control over the drugs. When he quit paying the mortgage Bett and I got evicted and moved in with her cousin, Lee. A few months later, Kelsey was born.

◆   ◆   ◆

I was watching TV one afternoon when I heard Bett yell from the bedroom, "Billy! Get in here! My water broke!"

I ran to her, trying not to act too nervous. I hadn't been around when Puff was born so it was all new to me. "What you want me to do?"

"Get me some clothes. Something to wear to the hospital. The baby's coming! Fast!"

I handed her a pair of her jeans and she threw them down on the floor and said, "Boy, are you crazy? I can't wear those. Get me a robe. What you thinking?"

"Oh," I said. "I just thought if it started coming out too soon the pants could catch …"

"Get my robe," she said, then mumbled something under her breath.

I drove her to the hospital and went to sit in the pink and blue waiting room. I talked to the other men for a few minutes, then got them to bet on whose baby would be born first; after all, it looked like Bett would barely be able to make it to the delivery room. We each put down ten bucks, and fifteen minutes later a nurse came to the door. I was half way out of my seat when she said, "Mr. Watson, you have a son. Please come with me."

Mr. Watson picked up the fifty dollars, smiled and thanked us all. After another two hours a different nurse appeared. "Mr. Hairston," she said, "you have a daughter."

When I walked into Bett's hospital room, her parents and sister were already there. None of them even looked at me. "What happened?" I said.

"Where you been?" Bett said. "Our sweet baby girl come into this world not five minutes after we got here."

"In the waiting room," I said, "where they sent me. But nobody told me nothing." *Shit,* I thought, *I could'a won that bet.*

"Where's the baby?" I asked. "I want to see my daughter."

"I'll take you," the nurse said, turning toward the door. "She's just beautiful." And she was right. Kelsey was beautiful.

◆   ◆   ◆

We took the baby home and continued to sell reefer and drugs. Puff, who was about five by then, started helping with the business. She'd sit at the kitchen table with me and help sort out the leaves and stems from marijuana, but her main job was to deliver to my dealers. I'd give her some reefer in a brown paper bag and she'd carry it into a house while I waited in the car. I put cocaine and heroin in baggies that I usually pinned under her clothing. I figured having a kid deliver the stuff would fool any cops who were watching me; they wouldn't think anything about a little girl running into a house for a minute. I never felt she was in any danger because she only delivered to the dealers who worked for me, and they were usually home with their own kids at the time. *She's safe,* I always thought to myself. *I'm right here to protect her.*

Within the next few years, the money started rolling in but Earl controlled everything and it rolled right on out again, for the most part. We must have been making fifty to seventy thousand dollars a year—in the 1980s when that meant something—and we bought everything we'd ever wanted: a nice split-level four-bedroom house, new furniture, cars, jewelry, and clothes. We traveled, sometimes taking Lee's family with us. We visited Disney World a couple of times and went gambling in Atlantic City and Las Vegas. We kept some of the old people in the neighborhood from being evicted from their homes, by paying their bills.

Once or twice I rented a bus and took Puff and Kelsey and their friends to King's Dominion Amusement Park. Another time I hired a local singing group for Puff's birthday. We bought uniforms and baseball equipment for one of the Little League teams.

I had a lot of juice in the community. That felt good. The people around me saw me as being successful. But there always had to be more, more, more. It was never enough. And I always had to be looking over my shoulder for the law.

In the 70s and 80s, selling drugs was like any other business; you competed with other dealers to get the most customers and make the most money. My regulars were often desperate and would do anything for drugs; women sometimes offered me their bodies, but I could never bring myself to use them like that. I often just gave them what they needed. Back then things were not as violent as they are today. After the appearance of crack, everything changed.

Heroin and cocaine addicts become mellow when they use the drugs. Crack addicts are much more active when they're using and seem to think nothing of killing a dealer they don't like. Today the dealers dress and act like gangsters; back in my day dealers were in a separate class from the users.

◆   ◆   ◆

One afternoon some of my dealers were at my house waiting for Earl to get there so we could start a meeting. As usual, they brought their kids along; there were always lots of children around, because we had all the latest toys. A couple of the dealers' girlfriends had come along with them, and they piled the kids, theirs and mine, into a car and took them to get ice cream while we talked. We were about to start without Earl when there was a loud pounding on the door and a deep voice shouted, "Police! Open up! Police! We've got a search warrant."

The cops came busting in, guns pulled, and ran toward us yelling, "Down! Get down on the floor! On your hands and knees!" We all dropped. Bett was in the bedroom with Kelsey, who was sleeping in the crib. The cops went from room to room, tossing stuff out of drawers, lifting up sofa cushions, looking under the beds; they must have searched for two or three hours. They finally found a little bit of coke that Bett had stuffed into Kelsey's diaper, but they didn't find the big stash we had hidden in the new washing machine.

Because Bett was listed as the owner of the house, she was arrested along with several of the dealers but they were all out on bond the same night. When the case later went to court it was dismissed. It set a precedent in Virginia law that stated that the owner of a dwelling could not be held accountable if a home did not have locks on the doors and others had free access to the premises.

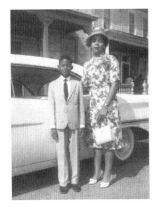
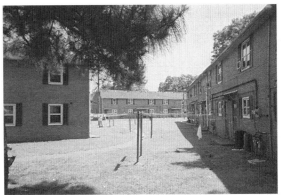

With my stepmother,
Cleo Hairston, about 1960

"Little Vietnam"—Portsmouth, VA
Life in the projects—before and after Vietnam

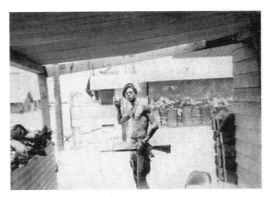

In Vietnam, 1970

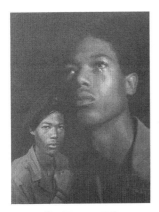

Viet Nam, 1970

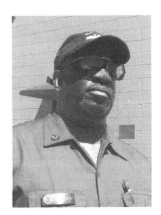

My Bro-Buck—friends for life

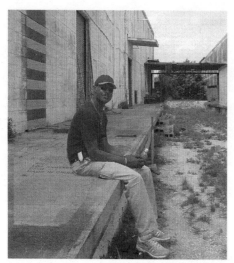

I moved from this place of residence in
Tampa, Florida on August 12, 1998

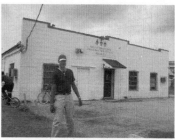

Where I signed up for Day's Work

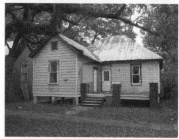

A Crack House

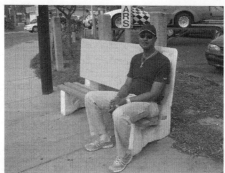

The bus stop bench where I waited to get into treatment, 1998

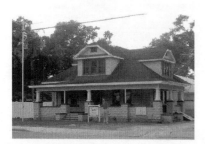

My last detox center, 1998

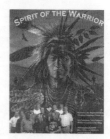

My PTSD Group's Poster, 1998

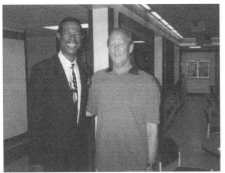

1st Year Anniversary of sobriety
with my first trusted friend, Patrick, 1999

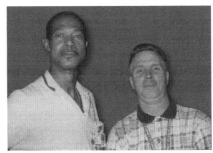

My first mentor, "Mr. C." 2000

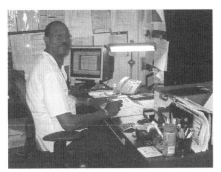

My office as Zone Manager 2000

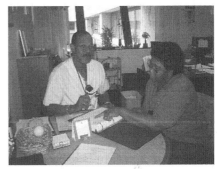

Working on a report with Carolyn
Burns Critical Care Work Leader
Specialist 2000

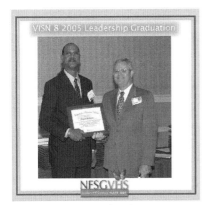

Receiving the
VISN Director Leadership Award
from Mr. George Gray, Jr. 2005

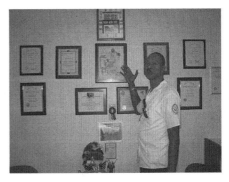

Wall of Achievement, 2006

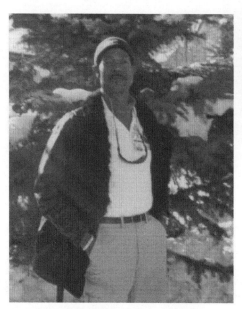

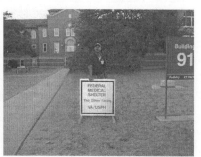

The Silver Lining Medical Shelter
for Katrina Hurricane Survivors,
Waco TX, 2005

Working security at the
2002 Winter Olympics
Salt Lake City, Utah

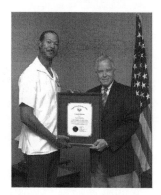

Receiving the National Hero
Award for work with
Hurricane Katrina survivors,
From W. Hopkins, Director 2006

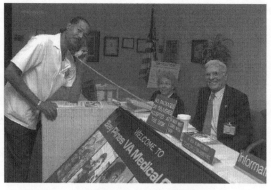

At work, Bay Pines Hospital
St. Pete, FL, 2006

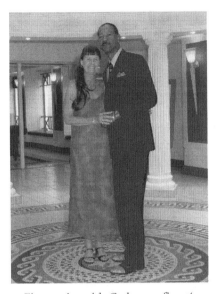

First cruise with Cathy, my fiancé

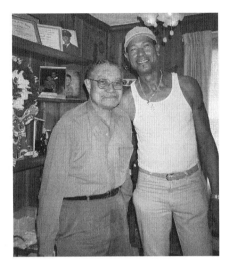

My Pop—who never gave up on me.

From the past—   To the present—

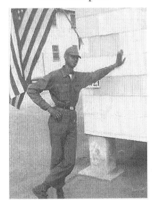

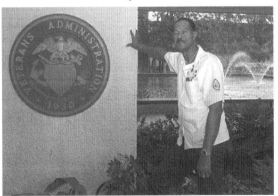

As a new recruit
Ft. Benning GA, 1969

Bay Pines V.A. Hospital
St. Pete, FL, 2006

Tied to the Bed

✦

1980–1986

It must have been six months later when I came in one night around midnight and was surprised to find nobody home. I was immediately filled with rage. I knew Bett had to be with that son of a bitch, Earl, and she'd probably left Puff and Kelsey with her sister or her mom. The more I thought about Bett and what she was doing, the more I drank, and the more I drank the angrier I got. I sat on the sofa all night watching television, waiting for her to show up. I thought over and over to myself, *She's my fucking wife and I don't deserve this kind of treatment. Goddamnit, I'm doing the best I can. All her running around is gonna stop. What I really should do,* I thought, *is just kill Earl.*

It was almost noon the next day when she came in alone. "Where the fuck you been?" I said.

She gave me a nasty look. "None of your goddamned business."

I stood up and followed her as she walked toward the kitchen. "What you mean, none of my business? You're my wife. And I know you been with Earl."

She opened the door to the fridge. "We wasn't doing nothing but bagging up some dope to sell."

"I know where you were," I yelled. "You was fucking Earl."

She whirled around and slammed the door. "You crazy! What do you care, anyway? All you want to do is get high."

I knew she was right. I couldn't stop. And I was ashamed of myself. "Bett," I said, "I know I keep breaking my promises, but …"

"You don't care about nothing but your dope. You ain't nothing but a thief and an addict." She went into the bedroom and just then the phone rang. I picked up the receiver.

"Billy? This Billy?" It was Lorretta, Earl's girlfriend, angry and crying.

"Yeah, this Billy."

"I know Bett just got home. 'Cause Earl just got home. That bitch been sleeping with my man and you need to beat her ass."

"Lor …"

"You should beat his ass, too," she screamed. "Beat both their asses." Then I heard Earl's voice on the phone, "Who is this? Who is this?"

I didn't answer, just hung up. A huge black rage welled up inside me. While we'd all known what was going on, nobody had ever said it out loud.

"Who's that?" Bett asked.

"Lorretta," I said. "She knows where you were." I grabbed my car keys and walked out, slamming the door behind me. I peeled away from the curb and broke the speed limit all the way to Lorretta's. She and Earl were on the front porch of the expensive apartment he'd rented for her, yelling at each other and jabbing the air with their fists while surprised neighbors stood around watching. Earl was trying to walk away when I ran up and grabbed him by the shoulders.

"You got something going on with Bett?" I shouted.

He pulled away and squinted his eyes at me, then he tried to get by me but I blocked his path. "I don't want to fight, man," he said in a calm tone. "Talk to Bett. I don't wanna fight."

Bett had followed me in her car and stood behind me shouting, "Earl, I love you!"

Lorretta yelled, "See, I told you, Billy! Kick his ass!"

I pushed him back and swung my fist at him. He ducked and grabbed me around the waist, pinning one of my arms to my side. With the my free hand I dug my finger into his eye, then hit him in the face, but he twisted away from me. He pulled out a pistol and aimed it at my chest. I saw the gun, but it didn't matter.

"I love you, Earl," Bett screamed. "I love you."

"I don't want to shoot you," Earl said to me. I raised my arms and had started toward him again when the gun went off. I felt a pain in my side. I didn't care. I still went after him, but he ran away.

People yelled all around us and the sound of a siren got louder and louder. While Earl raced around to the back of the house, Bett just stood there, looking after him. I got in the car about the time the police pulled up. "He's got a gun!" people screamed. "He's got a gun!"

They were talking about Earl, but the cops didn't seem to know that.

I raced away with a trail of police cars following. When I finally stopped ten or so blocks later, they surrounded me. With guns drawn, they shouted, "Get out of the car! Show your hands!" I didn't move. More cars pulled up, sirens blaring. "Get out of the car," they yelled on a bullhorn. "Show your hands! Now!"

I sat there, panicked, frozen, wishing they'd just shoot me and get it over with. My life wasn't worth living. *I'll be glad to die,* I thought. *Go ahead. Kill me.*

When one of the officers finally snatched the door open, he yelled at me, "You crazy? You could'a been shot! Why didn't you show your hands?" He dragged me out and they shoved me up against the side of the car and patted me down. "You're under arrest," he said. "Where's the gun?"

"Ain't got no gun," I said.

"We know you got a gun, asshole. Where is it?"

"Ain't got no gun. The other guy had a gun."

"You're under arrest, Jack. You're gonna be charged with eluding police and resisting arrest." They walked me to one of the police cars and shoved me in the back seat.

When we got to the police station, they started in again about where was the gun. I lifted up my shirt and showed them where the bullet had hit me. "Now you believe me? I ain't got no gun." The bullet wound had hurt, but what hurt more was Bett's saying that she loved Earl. That really hurt.

That incident and one other are forever burned into my mind. I came in one afternoon so high I could hardly find my way home. I threw myself down in a chair, where I kept nodding in and out. Bett was asleep on the couch and Puff and Kelsey were watching TV. I remember trying to focus on the kids' program but I couldn't stay awake. Puff, who must have been nine or ten by then, went in the kitchen and cooked up a can of Spaghetti. When she brought me a plate, even though I was out of it I remember her saying, "Daddy, please don't fall into your spaghetti." That statement slapped me right in the face. It told me that she knew what I'd become. I was so ashamed of myself. Puff's comment, and having Bett say that she loved Earl, not me, taught me a great deal about who I was. It was humiliating.

The next morning I was sitting at the kitchen table trying not to vomit, when Bett came in. "I can't keep doing this," I said. "You got to help me."

"Help you? I done everything I know how to do."

I looked up at her. "I got an idea," I said. "You can tie me up. Tie me to the bed so I can't get out and use no more."

"Just show me the rope," she said. "I'll tie you up all right."

And she did. We decided the kids shouldn't see what we were doing, so we told them they weren't allowed in the bedroom and closed the door. She tied my arms and legs to the bedposts, making sure the ropes were so short that I couldn't touch my hands together. It was uncomfortable, but once again, I hoped after three or four days of this I'd be through the worst part and would be strong enough to resist temptation.

She brought me meals and untied one of my hands so I could eat, then sat with me till I was done. When I needed to go to the bathroom she'd untie me and wait to tie me back up. It was about 10 p.m. on the second night when I called out to her and she didn't answer. I shouted her name over and over and finally Puff came and stood outside the bedroom door.

"Mama's not here," she said.

"Where'd she go?" I asked.

"I don't know. Said she'd be gone a few hours."

That did it. She was out seeing some man. I knew it. Immediately I was enraged. "Come in here, Puff," I said. "Open the door."

"But mama said not to open the door."

"I know." I did my best to sound calm. "But she's not here now and I need to use the bathroom."

"I don't want to make her mad."

"It's okay, Puff. I just have to use the bathroom."

After Puff untied me I told her she didn't have to wait, that I'd call her when I was done. I closed the door behind her and climbed out the window. Now I had a good excuse to get high.

◆   ◆   ◆

I kept dealing and life pretty much continued as it had. Bett still saw Earl but now all the secrets were out in the open. When my drug habit started costing more than $500 a day, I volunteered to go to the Rubicon Treatment Center in Richmond for eighteen months. They had a confrontational philosophy, where they said they'd tear you down and build you back up again. Nothing else had worked for me. I thought maybe it could help.

Rubicon was in a rundown residential neighborhood in Richmond. The ancient three-story brick building, surrounded by a tall chain link fence, was a remodeled elementary school. Bett drove me there, and as we pulled up in front of the building I said, "Now I'm still partners with you and Earl. Just because I'll be gone for a while, that don't change nothing."

Bett looked at me. "Nothing, except you ain't gonna be doing any of the work."

"I already got everything set up, you know that. And you can call me if you need me."

"Yeah, yeah, I know," she said, turning back to face the front.

"That's good," I said. "That's good." I got out of the car and she drove away.

During my first month at Rubicon I had to wear a piece of cloth that looked like a diaper over my shorts, and carry a baby bottle around because, they said, I needed rebirthing. I couldn't be alone.

There was a lot of in-your-face confrontation, both during the therapy sessions and outside them, from the counselors and from the other patients. It wasn't uncommon for people to break down under the pressure.

Leaving Rubicon without a pass was a serious infraction of the rules. One Saturday night, one of the women managed to sneak out and when they caught her coming back at 2 a.m., they decided to bring her up before the "family." It must have been almost 3 a.m. when they came through the dormitory, banging trashcan lids like they'd done in the Army, shouting, "Everyone to the media center, everyone to the media center."

They led us to a room that had candles lit all around it and the counselor said, "Sit down. We're having a funeral." Then the counselor said, "Someone sneaked out, and got high. Though she's walking, in reality she is dead. Dead to her family, to her friends, and to society." Then they rolled a casket into the room, with the woman who'd run away lying in it, crying. Some of us were assigned roles as her family members, friends and employers, and each of us walked around the casket, one at a time, and said what we thought that person would have said. We all acted as if we were crying.

"She was my wife," one of the guys said. "When we got married, she was so beautiful. Even my mom loved her."

"She was my mom. I don't know how I'm going to live without her," a woman said. "Mama, mama! Mama, don't leave me, please don't leave me. Now I cry myself to sleep every night."

"I was her aunt," one woman said. "She used to make peanut butter cookies for me and her mom, and was so proud of herself."

It was a powerful exercise, and affected many of us deeply. I began to realize how strong my addiction was and to understand that the possibility of dying from it was very real.

Some time later, because I'd been in Vietnam, the counselor suggested that I visit the Veteran's Center in Richmond. When I walked in the door of the place I was face-to-face with the big tree trunk my counselor had told me about. It looked like it was about four feet in diameter and maybe five feet high and was covered with names that had been burned into the smooth wood by veterans, honoring those they'd lost.

I picked up the wood-burning tool and knew immediately whose name I would leave there. It would be Doc, the medic who had reported the discrimination at our LZ before I got there, and who had disappeared without a trace. Although I hadn't actually met him, I knew he'd probably died from the same violent treatment I'd survived. As I burned the letters, D-O-C into the wood, I thought about him and the guys I'd served with in Vietnam. Tears came to my eyes. I remembered Slim telling me that Doc had written his mom every week, and she'd always sent him cookies that he shared with everybody. I'd been given a chance to live that he didn't have. It hit me hard. I owed it to myself and to him to do something good with my life. With a renewed sense of hope, I worked on my addictions and did my best to reach out to others.

In my last few months of treatment, my counselor made me a special "guru." If he had to leave a therapy group for some reason, I oversaw the rest of the session. I was told if I stayed clean for a year, I could come back and work at the treatment center. I was very proud of that.

A few weeks before I was to be released from Rubicon, Bett called me, crying. "You need to come home," she said between sobs. "You got to come back. Earl's dead."

"Dead?" I asked. "What happened?"

"He went to collect from our dealers," she said, pausing to catch her breath. "They set him up and jumped him."

"Bett …"

"They shot him, Billy!" She was screaming. "I'm scared. They may be after me! And the kids!"

"All right, all right. I'll be there tomorrow. I'll tell them that my cousin died and I want to go to his funeral." I went home but never planned to go to Earl's service. Even though he'd caused me lots of pain, I'd liked him and I was sorry he was dead. We'd been business partners and since I'd planned to keep dealing with him when I got out of treatment, I had to protect my interests. I got around and talked to people to let them know I'd be back soon, so they shouldn't get any ideas about taking over our territory because Earl was gone. Bett was involved, too, and I didn't want the competition to think they could get away with cheating her. I also felt that making sure others knew I'd soon be back would help to protect my daughters. When I got home I planned to sell drugs only until I had a good amount of money set aside, then I'd get into something legal. This time, I was going to stay clean.

The day before I was to go back to Rubicon, I went into the kitchen for something to eat and saw Earl's obituary notice lying on the table. When I read it and saw his survivors were listed as his relatives and a "very special close friend, Bett Hairston," instantly, a white rage flashed through me. I wadded up the paper and threw it across the room. I knew without any doubt, without any doubt at all, that she'd been fucking him while I was gone.

Then, I did the most natural thing in the world for me. The only way I knew to escape the pain. I went out on a binge.

When I was three weeks overdue at Rubicon, I was desperate to go back. The board agreed to let me return, but as a penalty I had to shave my head. I'd always been proud of the length of my hair, and I guess they thought it would help me get rid of any pride I might have left. I agreed. I'd have done anything. For the first week I had to "work my way back into the family," which meant spending ten hours a day scrubbing the steps with a toothbrush, or sitting in a corner facing the wall and not speaking to anyone.

This time I really tried hard to understand what the counselors were teaching, to stop comparing myself to others, to stop looking at the differences and instead start identifying the things we had in common. But, looking back, I now see that I didn't take any action, didn't change one thing I was doing. I wanted to "think right" and have that be enough. I wanted a simple answer that would solve all my problems. I told myself I just needed the right break.

In retrospect, I see that I already had those things. I got the right breaks but I threw those chances away. I was given a simple answer to make my life better. Just stop drinking and drugging. But it wasn't an easy answer. Definitely not the one I wanted. I could have tried to implement the principles I was taught in so many treatment centers that I lost count. But I didn't. I could have kept that job at the shipyard and eventually gotten on there permanently if I'd just kept my mouth shut. I could have held other jobs if I'd been a responsible employee. But I always listened to the wrong people, and the wrong voice in my head.

When I got out of Rubicon, I was back on drugs within a month. In spite of my determination to stay clean, I just couldn't do it. I was no longer in the drug business but I was around crack and coke all the time, and I couldn't resist. I'd gone from just selling to just using and soon all the money and business was gone. I was alone. Always alone. I was separated from everyone, trapped by a dark, overpowering fear.

I tried again to stop using. This time I found a job at a restaurant in Hampton, near Portsmouth. I thought if I stayed away from the old neighborhood, got away from my friends, that I could control my using drugs. I slept in an abandoned strip mall across the street from where I worked; I ate my meals and cleaned up at the restaurant. On Fridays I got paid and took the bus home. But as soon as I got back in Portsmouth, I went right out and bought drugs.

When I left that job I had nothing. Bett had lost the house and moved in with a new boyfriend. I moved around from here to there, living with my mom and Ivy until I couldn't stand the arguing and fighting anymore, staying with somebody else for a week or so, then moving to another friend's couch. For money, I stole and shoplifted at night. I was in my middle thirties and my entire life revolved around drugs.

I was miserable, an outcast, and still, I didn't get it. I did not understand that nothing would change until I did more than just think about it. I had to take some action to change it. Nothing changes till something changes.

◆   ◆   ◆

I was in and out of rehabs and jails, thirty days here, sixty days there, ninety days, six months, till I was thoroughly institutionalized and totally, completely without hope. When I got out, I found cooking jobs at small restaurants and kept shoplifting. I didn't see Puff and Kelsey for weeks at a time. Days and nights became a blur of misery and despair.

Eventually, I was sentenced to six years for possession of drugs. On my third trip to prison, I was sent to Camp 4 in the Shenandoah Valley, a two-hour drive from Portsmouth, far away from everybody and everything. It was a concrete building with heating and air conditioning, which was better than I'd had it before, and we could see three mountain ranges from there. I worked in the kitchen during what turned out to be a two-year bit. By this time I felt so bad about myself that I told my mom I didn't want her to visit me any more. But she and Bett always came anyway.

◆   ◆   ◆

I'd just finished cleaning up the cafeteria after dinner one night when one of the guys told me that my mom was on the telephone. She never called or wrote me, so I knew this couldn't be good. I went to the pay phone on the wall in the common area. I picked up the receiver and said, "Hello, Mom?"

"Hello, Billy Junior."

"What's wrong?"

"Your Aunt Lena died last night. Just thought you'd want to know."

I felt like someone had hit me in the gut. My head started spinning. *Oh, God. Oh, God. No. Not Aunt Lena.* My throat closed up. "What? What did you say?" I whispered.

"Lena died."

"Uh … uh … Why? What happened?"

"I'm not sure. Heart attack or stroke or something. Just thought I should tell you. I gotta go."

"But … but …" The line went dead.

I stood there with the phone at my ear, wanting to turn back time, to call my Aunt Lena and tell her I loved her. Finally, I took the receiver from my ear, looked at it, and hung it up. I couldn't let the other inmates see I was upset; I'd look weak and there would be a price to pay. I just stood there, clearing my throat till I thought I could talk. Then I asked the hack if I could be alone in the recreation area for a while. He nodded. I went out and sat down on a bench.

I leaned over, covered my face with my hands and sobbed. The only person who had ever cared about me was dead. Even though I hadn't seen her often in recent years, just knowing she was there had always given me comfort. I'd loved her more than anyone else in my life.

I cried because I'd lost her. Because my mother didn't love me. Because I was a disappointment to my father. Because I was a drug addict and an alcoholic. I cried because I was in prison, all alone. Because I was worthless. Because I couldn't support my family. I cried because Aunt Lena was gone and I was now really, completely, entirely alone in the world. I thought about her kindness and her strong faith and I thanked God for her. When I finally lay down on my bunk that night, for the first time in years, I went right to sleep and slept like a baby.

◆   ◆   ◆

When I got out of prison, Bett was living with another man. Just thinking about her drove me crazy. Once again, feeling betrayed and humiliated, I moved in with my mom and Ivy. I drank and drugged and felt sorry for myself, and for the third time suicide seemed the only answer. This time I slit my wrists, but once again my mom and Bett found me and took me to the hospital.

◆   ◆   ◆

A year or so later I got myself accepted into a treatment center in Hampton, Virginia, where for the first time I was to be treated for Post Traumatic Stress

Disorder (PTSD). After a group of us finished our initial paperwork, one of the counselors seated us in a large room, told us we were to watch a movie on PTSD and that he'd be back in twenty minutes.

The "movie" was actual film footage of a battle involving the First Air Cavalry, my old unit, and ground forces, fighting in Vietnam. The sounds of explosions, men screaming, the "whomp, whomp, whomp" of the choppers flying across the screen immediately jerked me back there. I was terrified. My heart raced and I broke out in a cold sweat. *No! No! Get me out of here!* I thought. *No!!* I was on fire with panic. I was stunned to hear that the voice of one of the dispatchers was mine.

It is! It's my voice I hear! That's me!

No, it can't be. I'm imagining things.

But it's true! It's my voice!

My heart was in my throat. Terror scorched every nerve in my body. I stood up shaking and walked out of the room and down the hall. The tremors were so bad I could hardly open the door. But finally, finally, I managed to get outside and I just kept going. Away. Away. Away.

After several tries, I got a cigarette lit and wandered around till I saw a bench at a bus stop. I sat down and stared straight ahead. I was numb. I seemed to be outside myself, not in my body. I was empty. Nothing was real. When the bus came, without thinking about it, I got on, and still in a daze headed home. I never even returned for my clothes.

Thirty days later I was back in jail.

My life went on like this for another two years, the same thing over and over and over. When any real problem arose, the only solution I could come up with was to use again. I always ended up right back where I started. Nowhere.

Mired in Despair

✦

1986–1998

Just released from another rehabilitation center, I was almost forty when I got a job at the Montgomery Ward in Virginia Beach. I turned out to be one of their most successful telemarketers and even managed to stay out of jail for six months. I was living at my mom's small place along with Ivy, her boyfriend, and her two children.

My mom had developed Alzheimer's Disease and sometimes she'd start cooking and forget what she was doing—once a frying pan full of grease caught fire but we were able to put it out. Other times she'd wander off and neighbors would bring her home. She was always fighting, attacking me and anybody else around. When she started hitting me, I'd grab her by the arms, take her to the bedroom, and lock her inside. It was the only way she ever calmed down.

"You need to take care of me," she'd scream at me. "I took care of you, now you got to take care of me. Ivy, she ain't doing shit. I hate her. I'm putting her outta this house." Then, when Ivy came home, my mom would go crying to her, saying Ivy was the only one who cared about her and how much she hated me.

I decided to try another geographic cure. When I asked the people in the personnel office at work if they could transfer me to another one of their stores, they suggested their offices in Tampa. Warm, sunny Florida sounded great. Before leaving, I made arrangements through the Veteran's Hospital in Hampton to go in for six months of drug treatment at the Tampa V.A. Then, when I was released, I'd have a job waiting at Montgomery Ward there. I even had a plan to get things cleared up with the law. I felt very responsible, making arrangements and getting organized.

I thought I only had to sign some papers and I'd be off parole but when I went to see my parole officer she said I'd have to come back the next day and take a blood test. I knew I wouldn't pass it and I also knew that would send me back to prison. I thought *Fuck it,* and borrowed enough money from Ivy to buy a bus ticket to Florida, plus another fifty dollars. Then I packed all my stuff in two suit-cases and a backpack, and went to the bus depot.

When I got to Tampa two days later, I was still coming down off heroin and shaking like crazy, so I went to the V.A. hospital. They admitted me to detox for a week, then referred to a place called Metropolitan Ministries for temporary housing.

As I left the hospital, I told myself this was the start of a new life in a new place. I could stay clean this time, for good. But when I got to the housing unit I wasn't so sure. I entered the yard of a three-story building, scattered with people sitting on flattened cardboard boxes and makeshift beds, protecting their trash bags of clothing and shopping carts filled full. It was easy to tell they were home-less by the filthy knapsacks, the dirty clothes, and the desperate looks in their eyes. I found my way to the door and rang the bell. They buzzed me in and I told the receptionist I'd been referred by my V.A. counselor for a three-month stay, the longest I could live there rent-free.

I called Montgomery Ward the next morning and they hired me right away. Then I called Ivy to let her know where I was staying, and I promised to stay in touch. She gave me Bett's phone number, and I called there and talked to Kelsey. I promised her, as well, that I'd let her know what was going on. Maybe some day she could even come down to visit, I said.

The first day on the job I impressed my co-workers by winning the award for having the most sales in a one-hour period, but I was careful not to get friendly with them because I didn't want them to know where I lived. On my lunch break I went outside and smoked cigarettes. I did my best to be optimistic and I stayed straight till my first paycheck.

That Friday I cashed my check at a convenience store and hung out on the street in front of Metropolitan Ministries. After a while I noticed some men standing around talking and when I heard the word "crack" I walked over their way.

"Hi, Brother," one of them said. "Name's Red." He was slim with reddish hair, had freckles all over his face, and a gold tooth. He looked very dirty.

"Hey, man. I'm Billy. Know where I can score some goods?" In a short time Red became my closest confidant. He got me what I needed, took me around the city and showed me the ropes.

I'd been doing telemarketing for two months when I was evicted from Metro-politan Ministries for staying out two nights in a row. For the first time in my life I was truly homeless. And I was scared. I ended up sleeping near Tampa's Port Authority, on Channelside Drive. The constant sounds from the ships docked there reminded me where I grew up, across from a Naval shipyard. I slept in overgrown vacant lots or in abandoned buildings. At that time, they were in the process of constructing the Florida Aquarium and the air was constantly filled with dust. I'd cough myself awake in the mornings to the sounds of the downtown traffic, the skyline of Tampa in the near distance. I ended up walking to and from work because I couldn't save bus fare. After six months I quit my job.

During the day I'd hang out on Nebraska Avenue with other homeless people and whores, where there was always a lot going on. Prostitutes sold themselves and drug deals were made in the rows of abandoned houses that were slated for demolition. Sometimes I'd walk down the railroad tracks hoping to find something that I could sell or trade for crack or food.

I started doing just enough day labor to get by and the rest of the time I sat around on the porches of abandoned houses, at bus stops or ball fields, thinking about what I had to do the next day to get more drugs and alcohol.

Living on the streets was chaotic. I was always alone. In the military and in prison I'd spent years in close, daily contact with a wide range of personalities from different backgrounds. In both, there were pretty clear regulations to live by. In the military good behavior was rewarded, while in the penitentiary good behavior was often penalized by the other prisoners as well as by the guards. But in both places, at least the rules were clear. Slowly, through harsh experience, I learned that living on the streets had its own loose set of rules.

There were several kinds of street people. Some, like me, lived on the streets because they had nowhere else to go. The truly homeless usually wore backpacks and sometimes pushed carts around filled with trash bags of their belongings. They worked and slept in the same clothing, seldom took a bath and earned what money they could from day labor. Those who received monthly disability checks from the government often rented a room for the first week or two of the month, but when their money ran out, they were back on the streets.

There were others, like Red, who actually had homes where they could live, but chose to hang out with the homeless. The word on the street was that Red's mother was a successful woman in a middle-class neighborhood, but Red wanted to be on the streets where he could buy and sell drugs. That type of "homeless" person would go home every few days to get a good meal, take a shower and get some clean clothes, then come back to the streets. Others were transients, running from town to town to escape the law.

All my life, I'd been able to talk to a person and get some sense of who that individual was, but it was very hard to do that on the streets. Every homeless person was isolated, imprisoned in his own little world of despair. Nobody trusted anybody else. Often I thought other homeless people were out to get me, and the paranoia from my drug use made it worse. I was afraid all the time. I was cut off from the rest of the world. Someone might pretend to be my friend and then while I was sleeping, take everything I had. If I let somebody know I had a little money from working day labor, they might get me high and beat me so they could take it. I most always stayed alone. I learned to never confide in anyone.

One night I broke into an abandoned house and fixed myself a place in a corner, thinking maybe I'd found a place I could stay for a while. But during the night three other homeless men came in and beat me up; a week later I heard about a man who was killed for doing the same thing I'd done, so I didn't do that again.

Sometimes I worked day jobs with a guy we called Smooth. He walked with confidence and was pretty laid back. He was well-built, looked like he worked out, had a gray-spotted beard and wore his hair short and nappy, which made him look dangerous. He always wore several layers of baggy clothing, even in the summer, and dirty tennis shoes. He walked fast, like he had purpose in his life, and didn't fly into rages as often as some of the other homeless men.

When I found work and got paid, I followed a regular routine. First, I'd go to a convenience store to cash my check and buy a fifth of wine and four or five quarts of beer, whatever was cheapest. Then, I'd go to a fast food restaurant hoping to find a "special," knowing that if I didn't eat before I started getting high, I wouldn't eat at all that night. The rest went for crack.

There weren't that many jobs on the weekends, and when I didn't work I didn't eat unless I found something in the garbage cans or the dumpsters behind restaurants. There was one place, Beef O'Bradys, where the cooks would sometimes put an entire meal out back in a Styrofoam container. Finding one of those was as good as my life got for the eight long years I lived on the streets.

◆   ◆   ◆

One Saturday morning, when I was back at Metropolitan Ministries, by then living in the chaos on the outside, I caught a break. Some guys looking for a day worker picked me out of the group to clean off a construction site for a new restaurant. I ended up working for them washing dishes for about six months. But I did more than just work in the kitchen; I became the restaurant owner's private drug dealer.

They moved me into the pool house behind the owner's home and I felt like I had it made. The room had a bed, a small sofa, a TV and a tiny cooking area. As soon as I could get to a phone, I called Portsmouth and talked to Kelsey, bragging that I was staying in a fancy place with a pool. She told me that Puff had a new baby boy, as well as all the other gossip; who had gotten married, who had died, who was working, and who was in jail. I told her I'd call once in a while to keep up on the family.

Gradually, the owner and I fell into a regular nightly routine. After I finished washing dishes and doing the salad prep, we'd go downtown where I'd score some drugs. Then we'd go back to the pool house and spend the night getting high with the manager and some other guys from the restaurant. In the beginning, he'd usually spend about a hundred dollars a night, but by the end I often scored nine hundred to a thousand dollars.

I found myself going for days, sometimes it seemed like weeks, without sleep. I lived in a thick fog, disconnected from the world around me. I was down to about one hundred and twenty pounds and since I'm six-foot-six, I looked like a walking skeleton. I was making three to four hundred dollars a week and just barely able to pay fifty bucks rent.

One night the manager gave me seven hundred dollars, plus twenty for gas, and sent me to score for him, driving his brand new Escalade. I wasn't feeling too good when I left and by the time I got to the crack house where I usually bought dope, I was dripping with sweat, had sharp pains in my stomach, and was really shaky.

The neighborhood was one of the most dangerous ones. The house was dark. I looked all around before I went up on the screen-enclosed porch and knocked on the door. Nobody answered. I knocked harder. "Hey in there!" I called. No response. I tried to look in the windows, but it was too dark to see anything. When I heard a noise behind me, I turned around.

"Hey," a deep voice said. "You looking for that girl who sells dope?"

"Yeah," I said, as he walked up to the porch and stood in the doorway.

"She ain't there," he said, pulling out a gun. "You can just give me your money."

"Hey, man," I said, fear blinding me as I held up my trembling hands.

"Now!" he shouted. "Gimme the fucking money!"

I pulled the cash from my pocket and threw it on the floor, thinking I'd run when he went for it. He reached over and picked it up, but I couldn't get around him to the stairs. "Is that all?" he said.

"I swear, man. That's all."

The man looked at me long and hard. "I just want to shoot you," he said.

"Hey, man, I'm cool," I said, holding up my hands that were shaking more than ever.

"Get off the fucking porch," he said.

I got by him and ran around the corner to the car as fast as I could. I knew if he saw the new Escalade he'd want to take that too, so I jumped in and got the hell outta there. All the way back I thought about how I'd tell the boss what had happened.

When I pulled up at the pool house he was sitting outside in one of the lawn chairs, waiting for me.

"Where's the stuff?" he said. "I need a hit. This whole day was fucked."

"I got robbed, man," I said. "I ain't got nothing."

"Where's my fucking money?" he shouted, getting up and coming for me. "I gave you seven hundred dollars, you son of a bitch. What did you do with my money?"

I held up my hands. "I told you, man. I got robbed."

"Gimme the fucking keys," he shouted, holding out his hand. I tossed them to him, and he walked toward the car. "This ain't the end of it," he said. "You gonna pay me back that money."

After I got my paycheck two days later, I caught the bus back downtown. I called them that night and told them I was going to Virginia and I'd come pick up my stuff some other time. No way would I ever even think of going back out there. So, I was on the streets. Once again.

In less than two days, I'd spent my whole paycheck. I returned to the day labor camps but since I'd been out of action for a while it was hard to get back to being the first one picked. Lots of days I went hungry. For another year and a half I survived somehow, doing day labor when I had to, chasing after drugs, living on the streets.

◆   ◆   ◆

One very good day I made fifty dollars on a construction job with Smooth and Red and some other guys. We pooled our money and bought some beer and wine and a whole lot of crack. Then we went to a row of abandoned homes that had "No Trespassing" signs posted all around them. We squatted on the upstairs porch of one of the houses so we could see the traffic below and were debating the nature of God when we heard voices and police radios. They were checking the houses. I hid the drug paraphernalia and we rolled up in blankets and acted like we were asleep, hoping they would think we were just a pile of blankets and mats on the porch.

But they busted us and we were all charged with trespassing. They ran checks on everybody and found I had an outstanding warrant in Virginia for parole violation, the "detail" I hadn't been able to take care of before coming to Florida. But I was relieved to hear that Virginia did not want to extradite me.

The judge gave me thirty days in jail with one year's probation. I didn't object. At least I'd be fed for a month. It wasn't bad; during most of my stay I had a cell to myself. I fit right in with the other prisoners.

The day of my release, I packed my clothes and my toothbrush along with an extra pair of underwear I'd stolen from the jail. Just before I was to leave, one of the guards came up and said, "Hey, Hairston. Chaplain wants to see you before you go."

Nothing Left

✦

1998

As I entered the Chaplain's office, he looked up. "Have a seat," he said.

I sat down across from him but he didn't say anything. Finally I said, "You wanted to see me?"

He leaned forward on his desk and folded his hands together. "I have some information for you," he said.

"What's that?" I asked.

"Your family in Virginia called a couple of weeks ago. Your mother died."

I sat there in silence, numb.

As the news started sinking in, my first reaction was guilt that I hadn't been there to take care of her. Then I wondered if Ivy had something to do with her death. After all, there were several life insurance policies that my mom had paid for faithfully, even when we had nothing to eat but beans. Finally, I thought, *She never loved me anyway. Why should I feel bad?*

Mostly I was dying for a drink.

"They left a number for you to call," the Chaplain said, pushing a small piece of paper across to me.

"This happened two weeks ago?" I asked, taking the number. "Why didn't you tell me about it then?"

"Well, the guards were concerned about how you might react."

I grabbed the paper, stood up and walked out. I had to get a drink. I could use the two dollars and fifty cents they'd just returned to me to take the bus several miles back to town, or I could buy a quart of cheap beer and a couple of cigarettes and walk.

As I trudged along sipping the Old Milwaukee, I felt relief for my mom; at least she'd no longer be suffering from Alzheimer's. Kelsey had told me a year before that the fighting between her and Ivy had gotten way out of hand and that

Kelsey had been appointed my mom's guardian so she could put her in a nursing home.

When I got in touch with Kelsey, she said I had to come up to sign papers because my mom had left a life insurance policy; a plane ticket was waiting for me at the airport and they'd meet me when I came in. The next day I made thirty-five dollars at a day labor job. Fifteen of that I had to give to my probation officer on my first visit to see her that same afternoon, but I was careful to save enough to get to the airport.

That night at the Salvation Army, I washed my T-shirt and jeans and took a shower. There was nothing I could do to improve the way my tennis shoes looked, but I did find a jacket to wear. The following day I flew home.

Nobody was there to meet me. I called Kelsey several times but never got an answer. Finally, I was able to reach Ivy, who came and got me. She said I could stay with her and her fourteen-year-old son and nine-year-old daughter. I was surprised at how old her kids looked.

Ivy was two months behind on her rent. I only had about six dollars. She had less than that, so we had to do something. I decided to ask my father to help us. For years, I'd only gone to see him to ask for something, usually money, and I hated the thought of doing it again. But this time I figured that since I'd be getting something from my mom's life insurance policy, I'd be able to pay him back. Maybe that would convince him.

I called Mama Cleo, my father's wife, and she invited me to come by and visit. I went the next day, embarrassed to be wearing such shabby clothes. Mama Cleo hugged me and invited me inside, and we walked back to my father's spotless study, just as we had the first time I'd met him when I was thirteen.

He looked up from the newspaper and said, "What were you in jail for this time?"

I felt my shoulders droop as the weight of his words pulled me down. I didn't answer.

"You ain't never gonna learn, are you? You got to do something about your life. You just got to stop drinking and drugging."

"I'm working on it," I said, "I'm trying. But right now things are really tight. I'm gonna need to borrow some money. Just enough to tide me over till the insurance money comes in, then I'll pay you back. We're signing the papers the day after tomorrow."

"Might have known," he said, pulling his chin in and looking up at me from under his eyebrows. "How much?"

"Maybe three hundred," I said. "Ivy's behind on her rent. They said it could be six or eight weeks before we get the insurance money. And I'll get a job."

"And you gonna pay it back." he said.

"Yes, I will. I sure will. I'll have plenty of money in a few weeks."

He looked over at Mama Cleo, then back at me. "All right. Three hundred. But I'm expecting every penny of it back," he said.

"Thanks, Pop," I said. "You won't be sorry."

The next day Mama Cleo came and picked me up. She said, "Your daddy didn't like the way you were dressed. We're gonna get you some decent clothes." She bought me pants and a shirt, a jacket, and a pair of dress shoes.

Since Kelsey was my mom's guardian, she went down with Ivy and me to sign the papers at the funeral home the next day. Although my mom hadn't missed an insurance payment in twenty-five years, when she went into the nursing home, payments were not made on two of the policies, and they lapsed. When we called about them, the insurance companies insisted there was nothing they could do about it. However, the third policy was still in effect, and after all the bills were paid, Ivy and I were each to receive about eight thousand dollars.

Two weeks later, after we'd spent all the money Pop had lent me on drugs, Ivy was evicted and we all moved to a filthy fleabag motel that catered to prostitutes. Ivy and the kids slept in the bed and I spent the nights on the floor or in a chair. We boosted to get money for food and drugs, but there was never enough. Finally, I went back and asked my father for another loan. This time he said no, but Mama Cleo slipped me a little when he wasn't watching.

Three months later, when the insurance checks finally came in, Ivy and I went on a drug spree. I got this brainstorm to return to Florida for a couple of days, where crack was really cheap, buy some, and bring it back to Virginia to sell. My next brilliant idea was to take only one thousand dollars of my share of the money with me, and leave the remaining seven with Ivy. Before I left I told her that I owed my father and Mama Cleo three hundred dollars and she said she'd see to it that they got the money. Of course, she didn't.

In Tampa, I rented a room in a trashy motel that was close to some of my old crack houses. I found Red and Smooth and told them my great plan, bought some drugs and went on another binge. As I started coming down from each high I wanted more and more, and for once I had the money to get it. But along with the drugs came a paranoia so strong that I locked myself in the room and couldn't leave, even for food. When I ran out of money I called Ivy, but she had disappeared with all of it.

Broke again, within a week I was back on the streets. I was still paranoid and desperate, sure that somebody was out to kill me. After finishing a job late one afternoon, I bought myself a six-pack and some wine, and crawled into my raggedy refrigerator box behind an abandoned building near downtown Tampa.

Listening

✦

1998

On the morning of August 12, 1998, I woke up in that box just as a security guard approached. He ran me off, as others had done many times, and I stumbled down the street where I sat down on the curb and held my head in my hands. A quiet voice in my head said, *I need to change my life.*

For decades, every morning I got up thinking that I had to stop drinking and drugging. Or get out of trouble. Or find a job. Or earn some money. But this was different. It came from a different place within me. For the first time I really listened to the voice that had always been there.

I called my V.A. representative who managed to get me into a detox center that same day, which surprised me. When I arrived there at 10 a.m. they told me I'd have to come back at 5 p.m. Since I had nowhere else to go, I sat on a bus stop bench across the street from the building. The last time I'd eaten was the day before when I had a bologna sandwich. I was dying of thirst.

After a while, a man carrying a tall Budweiser in a small brown paper bag sat down beside me. I heard the metallic "pop" as he opened the can. Just then, the bus pulled up and when he walked toward it, the driver signaled that he couldn't bring the beer with him. He returned to the bench and put the beer down beside me. He got on the bus. He had not even taken a sip of the beer.

I stared at the can. My head throbbed as I lifted my shaking hand and wiped sweat from my brow. My mouth was dry and my stomach ached from hunger. The beer was still so cold that the paper bag was wet with condensation. I looked at the treatment center and I looked at the beer. I looked back at the treatment center and again at the beer.

I can drink just one, I thought. *Then I'll go on in for treatment …*
No, if I drink one, I won't stop. I'll end up back downtown and I'll die …
Only one beer … What's one beer gonna hurt?

Without making any conscious decision to do it, I saw my trembling hand reach out toward the beer.

I tipped it over.

I watched the cold pale liquid foam and splash to the sidewalk. I smelled its sweet odor. Then I stood up and walked away.

As I headed up the street I saw a twisted old grapefruit tree in a vacant lot. I pulled off a small piece of fruit, clearly not yet ripe, and my stomach growled as peeled it. A violent shudder ran through my body when I sucked the sour, bitter taste into my mouth. But I was so hungry and thirsty I kept eating. It seemed to me to be a gift from God.

I found a cigarette butt to smoke, and as I started walking around the block I looked down at my feet, appearing and disappearing under me, one at a time. I walked and I walked and I walked. I thought about my mom, whose approval I could never get, always saying I'd never amount to anything. I remembered Aunt Lena. In my head, I could see her smiling at me.

I thought about the path I'd started on in high school, drinking and smoking reefer. I saw how addiction had led me to Vietnam, to prison, and finally to the streets; how it took over my entire family. I was exhausted, disgusted with myself. I had no pride. I couldn't fake it anymore. Finally I was ready to DO something, to take some action. I thought this way before, many times before, but this time it felt different.

When I walked in the door of treatment center at 5:00 that day, the only things I owned were the pants, shirt, and shoes that Mama Cleo had bought me while I was home a few months before. I'd long ago abandoned underwear. All I carried was a raggedy backpack that held a comb and an ink pen. I was covered with dirt and sweat and I knew how bad I smelled.

I was welcomed at the treatment center and they suggested that the first thing I needed to do was to take a bath. They had no clothes I could borrow, but they offered to let me use the washing machine. While my pants and shirt were sloshing around in warm soapy water, I took the first hot shower I'd had in weeks. They gave me two hospital gowns to wear; I put one on backwards and the other on frontward, stepped into my smelly shoes and went to the first AA meeting where I really listened to what was being said instead of thinking about what I would say. For the very first time, I stopped comparing my story with other people's lives and instead, started identifying with their thoughts and feelings. I stopped trying to decide whether I was an alcoholic or a drug addict. In reality the label didn't matter. I was a child of God.

As I sat in that room, just skin and bones, shaking from withdrawal and shivering in the air conditioning, I heard in a new and different way that there was a solution that had worked for countless people and that it could work for me. I'd heard those words before, but this time I clearly understood them. I heard concrete suggestions being offered to others and decided to put those ideas to use in my own life, things that I could practice daily.

That night as I tossed and turned in bed, first cold, then hot, I kept praying to God to please help me. Memories of AA meetings I'd attended in years past and people I'd met in rehabs kept flashing through my mind: Doc and the guys in Vietnam, the people at the Rubicon Treatment Center, the old timers at so many AA and NA meetings who tried to get me to listen to them.

I'd always thought those people who had told me to pray, or to face my fears, or to live one day at a time were hypocrites because when I made half-hearted attempts to follow their suggestions, I never got any results. I knew recovery and rehabilitation programs inside and out, understood the dynamics behind the suggestions, and had "talked the talk" for years. I could explain the process to anyone who wanted to know. For the first time I realized that I'd never once really tried to *live* by the steps. I now think it didn't work because I completely ignored the fact that *action* was the key. I tried to think myself into right action instead of taking action that would lead me to right thinking.

As my week in detox was coming to a close, my V.A. rep. found me a bed in a treatment center called Turning Point. When I arrived, the staff there explained that there wouldn't be a bed available for the first three nights, but after that I'd share a room with one other man. I was more than happy to sleep on a mattress on the floor.

From the beginning, I went to all of the Twelve Step meetings they had, Narcotics Anonymous, Alcoholics Anonymous, Cocaine Anonymous, and would have attended anything else that was offered. The one that hooked me was AA because of the love and hope I felt there.

When I'd been at Turning Point for a few weeks, I began to see changes in myself and started believing that maybe I could become the man I'd always wanted to be. Although it seemed to me that some of the others still looked at me as if I was scum, in the AA meetings I felt accepted for the first time since I could remember. Those conducting the meetings told stories about themselves that I could relate to; their thoughts and fears were the same as mine. They shook my hand and hugged me and told me to keep coming back.

I started remembering things I'd heard when I was bouncing in and out of the rooms of AA, from as far back as the days when I went to meetings just to get out of the cell block and have some coffee and cookies. I'd been told to go to the meetings early, to help set things up and to get involved, to live one day at a time, and to keep it simple.

At Turning Point, patients were assigned duties each week. Even when my assignment was in the kitchen or sweeping up the dorm, I also helped arrange the chairs and tables for meetings and took them down afterwards. And at every meeting I sat in the front row and was always careful to thank the chairperson.

I often sat next to a young lady who seemed to think the Twelve Step Programs had a hidden angle. After every meeting she'd offer me a cigarette and we'd sit on a bench in the hall and talk about things we'd just heard. One night she looked at me from the corner of her eye and said, "Did you catch 'em yet?"

And I said, "Naw, I didn't catch nobody. Catch 'em what?"

"Did you catch 'em?" She turned to face me.

"I don't know what you mean."

"It can't be as simple as what they're saying." She lit a cigarette and blew the smoke out the side of her mouth. "There's got to be a secret. And I'm going to keep going to meetings, and sooner or later somebody will slip and I'll find out the secret."

I laughed, but deep down I said to myself that maybe she was right, so I kept going to the meetings too, because if there was a secret, I didn't want to miss it. But I learned that there is no secret. It's a simple program. It may not be easy, but it's simple. But you have to take action and make changes to work it. Without action, nothing happens.

While I was at Turning Point, a V.A. representative from the Bay Pines Hospital in St. Petersburg came every Thursday to talk about their programs. The ones that most appealed to me were the Substance Abuse Treatment Program (SATP) and the Compensated Work Therapy Program (CWT), where I could be employed at the hospital after I finished treatment, and save money to get a place to stay. A week before I was to be released from the Turning Point, I got the V.A. rep to schedule a meeting for me to make an application.

Starting from Scratch

♦

1998

I rode the bus from Turning Point to Bay Pines Veteran's Hospital in St. Pete early the next Tuesday morning, wearing my best clothes: cut off shorts, a shirt I'd gotten from the Turning Point clothing room, and the dress shoes Mama Cleo had bought me. I hated having to wear the shorts; since I was down to about a hundred and twenty pounds, my legs looked like toothpicks and I felt like everybody was looking at me.

All the way there I worried about getting turned down. I was terrified I'd end up back on the streets. It would be a death sentence. I imagined the social worker saying, "Sorry, Mr. Hairston, we just don't have room for you. We need to give our beds to people who deserve them."

I entered the spotless hallway of a one-story domiciliary behind the main hospital building, as I'd been directed. A bell rang when I opened the door to the reception room and within a few moments a woman came in, took my name and told me to have a seat. Three others were waiting, and I nodded to them and sat down. All I could think about was how, if this didn't work out, I'd end up living in a cardboard box again. And I knew I'd die out there.

After about twenty minutes a counselor asked me into her office, which was cluttered with manuals, books, stacks of papers and photos of herself with three children. She went through my file while I sat there, then looked at me over the top of her glasses.

"You've spent eight years living on the streets?"

"That's right," I said. "Eight years."

"I see here that you were diagnosed with PTSD at the Hampton V.A. Did you ever receive any treatment for it?"

"No, I haven't. Every time I've gone to the V.A., when I told the doctors I had a drug problem, that's all they paid attention to. I got drug treatment and that's it."

"I see," she said.

"Early on, I learned that treatment for PTSD was offered only to those who had been in direct combat or who had been wounded," I said. "Even back then you had to say you were crazy or they just gave you drugs."

She flipped through the file, stopping to go over something here and there or to ask a question. I tried to read her face, to find the hidden meaning in the tone of her voice, to figure out what she was thinking, what my chances were, but I couldn't tell anything. The thought of being turned away sent me into a panic. I heard that voice in my head again telling me that the beds were needed for those who deserved them. Tears filled my eyes.

She handed me a tissue and said, "Although we usually start patients out in treatment for addictions, I believe that program is full right now, so I'm going to recommend that you enter our PTSD Program first. It's clear that you're under great stress, and your file shows a long history of the symptoms of PTSD. It's not only from Vietnam; it's also because you've lived on the streets for so long."

I cleared my throat. "That's good. Thank you. Thank you."

"I'll need to take a minute to go check on some things." She looked at me steadily. "What would you be willing to do if I can get you in?"

"I'll do anything and everything you tell me. It doesn't matter what it is, I'll do it. But please don't send me back out there. Please!" I was begging, and again the tears started flowing fast.

She came around the desk, patted my shoulder and said, "I won't send you back. I know there's a waiting list, but maybe we can get around it." Then she left.

I'm going to get in, I thought. *They're going to take me.* I covered my face and cried out loud, overwhelmed with relief. While I waited, I prayed as hard as I could that she'd be able to find an opening. I promised God that this time I'd make it. I'd do whatever it took. No matter how hard it was, I wouldn't give up. I'd reached the end of the road.

When the counselor returned she wasn't smiling. "Mr. Hairston," she said, sitting back down at her desk, "I'm sorry to tell you it doesn't look good. I've checked with the PTSD program to see if we could give you priority, but they want you to get addiction treatment first." A heavy blanket of hopelessness smothered me. I couldn't breathe.

My bottom lip quivered. I slumped forward and covered my face, trying to get control of myself, but despair consumed me. I sobbed into my hands in misery. I couldn't stop.

She came from behind her desk and touched my arm. "I'm sorry," she said, handing me more tissues.

I took the tissues and blotted my eyes. "If I can't get in here," I said, trying without success to keep my voice steady, "I'll end up … back on the streets … And that means … I'm going to die." I looked directly at her. "The last time I was this scared … I was in a helicopter in Vietnam … and somebody was … trying to kill me."

She reached over her desk and picked up my file. "Let me give the SATP Program a try, Mr. Hairston. We're not going to send you back to the streets. I'll find something." She left the room again, and I sat there, numb. I was afraid to hope it would work out, and afraid not to hope. I was staring death in the face. After an endless wait, she came in with a big smile on her face. She sat down and said, "I couldn't get you into the PTSD program right now, but I did find a place in the SATP where you can get help with your addictions. And you can come in today. It's a start."

I can't begin to describe the relief I felt. You're talking about a guy … I'd never been so happy to be institutionalized in my whole life. And drug treatment was what I'd wanted to start with, anyway. When we finished the paperwork I ran all the way to the bus stop, rode back to Turning Point, where I grabbed my stuff and caught the next bus back to the hospital. Looking out the window as we drove through the city, I saw people walking on the sidewalks, normal, happy people with everyday lives. I wondered if I could ever be like them.

I felt hope for the first time since I could remember. Then it occurred to me that for the first time ever, I was going to treatment because I really wanted to, not to run away from other drug dealers, or to escape my unbearable life, or stay out of prison.

◆   ◆   ◆

There were twenty-four men at our first SATP meeting, most looking depressed or angry. A few were in cut-off shirts and jeans and several wore leather jackets. Some had bandanas wrapped around their heads. We ranged in age from our thirties to our sixties; two of us were Vietnam vets, one was from the Gulf War and one from the Korean War. The rest were peacetime soldiers and we were from all branches of the service, the Army, Navy, Marines and the Air Force. One was a successful businessman, two of us were homeless, and most of the others were there because they were about to lose their jobs or their families.

First, the Program Clerk told us the rules and regulations. We couldn't leave the campus during the month we were in treatment, but we could attend AA meetings that were brought in to the hospital by alcoholics from the outside. He took us on a tour of the floor where we'd be living for the next four weeks. Two men shared each of the bedrooms and there were several group therapy meeting rooms, as well as offices for the psychologist and psychiatrist. There was also an area with chairs and a television where we could relax at the end of the day, when we weren't doing homework assignments like reading, writing, or working on a hobby.

The male nurse practitioner took each man's medical history and gave us all physical exams. He explained that he'd be passing out our medications twice a day. Each of us would see a psychologist for individual therapy, a psychiatrist once a week, and have ongoing individual or group therapy three or four times a day.

When he gave me my physical, he found a lump by my jaw that I hadn't even noticed. As he touched it and tried to move it around, he got a worried look on his face. "How long have you had this?" he said.

"Had what?" I asked him.

"This lump. This concerns me," he said.

"I don't know," I said, reaching up to touch it. "Didn't know it was there."

"Were you ever injured in that area?"

"Years ago I got hit with a baseball bat, but I never went to the doctor or anything."

"We need to check it out," he said, stepping back and looking me in the eye. "It's probably benign, nothing to worry about, but we'll get it taken care of soon as you finish the SATP."

I was struck by his compassion and the fact that he talked to me as if I was as good as anyone else, instead of just some nameless homeless person. It had been a very long time since anyone had shown an interest in my welfare.

The following day I had my first session with my counselor, Rick. I wasn't looking forward to telling my story again. I'd been through it all so many times in so many rehabs—I dreaded having to drag it out once more.

He was walking out of his office as I came in, and he said, "Just move those papers off the chair and have a seat. I'll be right back." The room had one small, high window and the walls were covered with diplomas and plaques. There were two cushioned chairs, one blue and one aqua, and a beige studio couch. Books, magazines, files, and papers were stacked everywhere, most with post-it notes sticking out of them. I moved a stack of books and sat down in the aqua chair.

While I waited for him I recalled the times I'd sat in other chairs like this, hoping somebody could fix me, get rid of my addictions for me. But this time I knew that if I wanted this to work I had to be the one to do something different. I had to be completely honest. This time I could leave nothing out.

Rick rushed back in a few minutes later, closed the door and reached out to shake my hand. He smiled. "Rick Keathley. Sorry for being late. This place can get crazy." He was stocky, had light brown hair but was bald on top and wore wire-rimmed glasses. He wheeled his chair around from behind his desk and sat down, facing me.

"That's okay," I said.

He picked up a file and looked at the tab. "Okay, Eugene. Eugene Hairston, right?"

"That's right."

"Okay. So, first off, let me tell you that I've read your file, and I want you to know that I'm an ex-addict and a Vietnam vet like you."

"That sounds good," I said. "Well, not good, but I know you can relate to where I've been."

He looked through the file. "Your mom is dead but your dad is still alive. Is that right?"

"That's right."

"And I see here you're married with two daughters. None of your family lives in Florida. Right?"

"That's right."

"And now long have you been using?"

"Since I was thirteen or fourteen years old."

"Okay now," he said, closing the file. "Do you have any questions for me before we get started?"

"No. None I can think of. But there is one thing I want to tell you."

"All right," he said. "Go ahead."

I didn't want to tell on myself, but I knew I had to. I looked down at the floor. "Well, I, um, I've been in lots of treatment centers."

"Yes, I know. It's in your file."

"And I was always good at following the rules. I knew how to make myself look good."

"Okay."

I looked up at him. "But the truth is, I was just saying what people wanted to hear. I made a list of things I wished I hadn't done, but I left out the worst ones. I said I'd made amends to people I'd harmed, but I hadn't.

"And now you realize you were only cheating yourself?"

"Yeah, man. That's right. I always planned to go back to selling dope as soon as I got out and most of the time I'd planned to go back to using, too, thinking I'd be able to control it. It's the only way I knew how to support myself. But in every treatment center the counselors said they'd seen a change in my attitude and behavior and they felt I had an excellent chance of staying clean."

"I see."

I looked at him. "I never once really tried to work the program, to 'walk the walk,' I just 'talked the talk.' And I always went back to using. I want you to stop me if you see me trying to fake it. I don't want to fail no more."

He looked me dead in the eye. "You don't have to fail again," he said.

For some reason, I believed him.

He grabbed a pen and notebook. "Okay, let's start at the beginning. Tell me about yourself and your family, everything that comes to mind. What was it like for you growing up?"

Mean Aunt Ro

✦

1998

I took a deep breath and leaned forward, thinking to myself, *Here we go again. One more time.* "The beginning. I was born in Portsmouth, Virginia, in 1951. My real name is Eugene but I was called Billy Junior while I was growing up, after my father. In Vietnam they started calling me Treetop."

"All right, Treetop."

"My parents split up when I was a baby and I don't remember seeing my father till I was a teenager. I was sick a lot and when I was four I went to the hospital. I remember it clear as yesterday. I woke up and my mom was sitting in a chair beside the bed, wiping her eyes. I'd never ever seen her cry before and that scared me. She'd get mad and yell and scream and fight, but she never cried. She wiped her cheeks, cleared her throat, and said, 'Billy Junior, the doctors say you're real sick. They ain't sure they can make you well.' She patted my arm. 'But they're going to try, baby.'

"I was just glad she stopped crying. 'It's all right, Mama,' I said. 'I'll be okay.'

"She said it was gonna be up to God. I remember thinking that God probably didn't even know I was alive."

"So the fact that your mom was crying scared you?" Rick said.

"Damn right it did," I said. "If she was crying something was really wrong—that meant there was something she couldn't fix, and that just didn't happen. She could be really tough. And if she was scared then I was scared. Anyway, they decided I had sickle cell anemia and for a couple of years I had blood transfusions every month. But even with the treatments, I got a lot of colds and was as skinny as a rail. My mom was always feeling my forehead and saying, 'Shit. You coming down with something again. You need some medicine.' Then she'd give me her favorite remedy, rock candy with gin. Even after I stopped having the transfusions I stayed very thin. I always felt ugly, just skin and bones with my big ears sticking out. I was sure nobody could ever love me. I sure didn't love me."

"That must have been hard."

I felt tears starting up, but I couldn't cry now. We'd hardly gotten started. I cleared my throat.

"How do you think the illness affected you?" he asked.

"Well, I missed a lot of school. And I watched a lot of TV, which I felt was a lot better than going to school." My mind went back to our old place in Portsmouth. "I must have been about seven or eight when we got our first TV set. We couldn't afford to buy one, so my mom rented a 'Meter-matic.' It was a great big thing with a little six-inch screen and it had a gray meter box attached to the side. When we put a quarter in the slot we could watch for a half-hour. That got expensive pretty fast, so I found a way to insert the tip of an old butter knife till the TV switched on. Then I watched all the shows I wanted." I laughed again and Rick joined in.

"My favorite was the 'Morning Movie.' As it came on, they showed a steaming cup of coffee and a lit cigarette sitting in an ashtray. I'd always make me up some coffee and get one of my mom's cigarettes, then settle down on the sofa. It made me feel all grown-up and safe. That was great till the man who collected the coins realized that they weren't making any money on us and took the TV back."

"Sounds like you learned early on how to take care of yourself."

"Guess I did, in some ways."

"Let's go back to the sickle cell. Did the transfusions help?"

"I was okay for a while, but when I was eight I ended up in the hospital again with stomach pain. One memory stands out. I was in a dark ward with lots of empty beds; as I recall, the only light in the room was the one right over my head. I was asleep when my mom and my Aunt Lena arrived along with some of the church sisters, but when I felt a cool hand on my forehead I knew it was Aunt Lena. She was my favorite aunt. Actually, she was my favorite person in all the world." It felt good just thinking about her. I smiled and nodded my head.

"I opened my eyes. She was standing over me, blotting her face with a handkerchief. She always sweated when she prayed, and I knew why she was there. She was a great big woman, dark-skinned, and she wore long dresses covered with big flowers. When she walked, her skirt waved like a flag, but she moved fast and when us kids went somewhere with her we had to run to keep up. She had little black moles like freckles all over her face and when she laughed, which she did all the time, her cheeks looked like small balloons. You couldn't help but laugh with her."

Rick shifted in his seat and made a note on the legal pad he was holding.

"Anyway, back to the hospital. Aunt Lena said, 'Billy Junior, now, don't you pay us no mind. You just go right on back to sleep, Honey. Your mama and Aunt Lena and the church sisters, we're all here and we're gonna to pray for you. And God'll answer our prayers. All you gotta do is believe.' I heard the sisters in the background, saying softly, over and over, 'We believe,' and 'Praise Jesus,' and 'Thank you Jesus.' I don't know if I believed in God back then, but I believed in Aunt Lena.

"I don't remember this part, but later on Aunt Lena told me that the next morning I was so much better that the doctors were confounded. The doctors may have been confounded but she wasn't. She never doubted it was a miracle. It was like her little secret that the doctors didn't understand what had really happened."

"Your Aunt Lena sounds like quite a woman," Rick said. "Somebody you could count on. Was she your mom's sister?"

"No. Aunt Lena and her brother, Uncle James, weren't really our blood relatives. They lived with my mother's family when they were kids. My mom said their folks kicked them out because Lena was too fat and James was too dark-skinned. But my Aunt Peggy, now she *was* my mom's sister, she told me that where they grew up down south, things like that happened all the time. If a family was having a hard year, one or two of the kids might stay with a family who was doing better. But whatever, when I was little those two were the most generous people in my life. Their smiles and their hugs told me they loved me, and I was sure they were the only ones who did."

As I thought of Aunt Lena, the warm, safe feeling I always had with her came back. I felt like she was sitting beside me, encouraging me. I looked up through Rick's high office window, to the blue sky outside, remembering. "Aunt Lena always had something on the stove for us, maybe biscuits and fried fat back, that we called 'stick o' lean, stick o' fat.' Or maybe she'd have sausages and corn bread. We drank Kool-Aid with sugar, Kool-Aid without sugar, and sometimes, just water sweetened with a little sugar. Every time Aunt Lena saw me she'd open her arms wide and say, 'There go my Billy Junior. Come here boy, and give Aunt Lena a hug.' And when I squeezed her neck she'd shout, 'Oh, he's so strong, boy.' She'd pick me up and twirl me around and tickle me till I screamed with laughter and tried to wiggle away." I paused, thinking. "Today I believe it was my Aunt Lena's prayers that kept me alive through my most desperate years."

Rick said, "You know, it's important for every child to have at least one adult who believes in them. Maybe she was that person for you."

"She was," I said. "She was for sure."

"What about her brother?" Rick asked.

"Uncle James lived in New Jersey, but when I was little he visited us every year. He was huge and muscular, very dark-skinned and he laughed all the time, showing his mouthful of gold teeth. He laughed just like Aunt Lena. He was a mechanic and drove a long distance tractor-trailer. I don't know where Uncle James got all his cars, but every summer he showed up with a different Cadillac.

"He'd pick me up and say, 'My, my, my. Who is this tall, handsome young man? Them ears getting bigger or is that face getting smaller?' Then he'd laugh and laugh. And he never forgot to bring me a present. My favorite was a jungle outfit. I used to have a picture of me in my safari hat, holding a rifle and wearing a tool belt that—now let's see if I can remember it all—it had a pistol, a flashlight, handcuffs and bullets, the works! I was so proud of that rifle. There I was in that picture, standing in front of his latest Cadillac with my ears sticking out farther than the brim of my safari hat. I always loved seeing Uncle James. Until he married Aunt Ro."

"You didn't like her?" Rick asked.

A cloud of dread fell over me when I spoke her name. "She didn't like me! My mom sent me to stay with them the during summer vacations when I was eleven and twelve. Uncle James was glad to have me there but Aunt Ro always treated me like the poor relation I was. She told me I had to pay my way by cleaning the house and doing whatever else she wanted. I was just there to wait on her.

"Tell me about her."

"She was just mean. She was short and heavy, had a small mustache and always wore her hair in a tight little bun, which made her jowls stand out. She wore loose colorful dresses, always with the sleeves rolled up which showed her short arms and fat fingers. She had a gold tooth that could be seen on the rare occasions when she smiled."

"Did your Uncle James defend you?"

I didn't want to answer—to say out loud that Uncle James had abandoned me, too. But he had. I reminded myself to be honest. "He didn't say nothing. Just let it go on. I could never understand that, big man like him. He couldn't have been afraid of her."

"You sure about that?" Rick asked.

I looked at Rick and shook my head. "I don't know why he didn't stand up to her because I always felt like he cared about me. When it was just the two of us, it was great. I don't know what to tell you. It don't make sense to me.

"Anyways, during my second summer with them, their boys were little, maybe three or four years old, and their daughter, Alyvia, was about eight or nine. I'd been there only a couple of days when Aunt Ro said she was taking her kids to a movie, and while they were gone I had to clean the bathrooms. That made me feel so low, like I was a servant or something. But all I said was, 'Yes, ma'am.'

"She was always saying hateful things." I put a sneer on my face, mimicking her, "'We hardly got the money to feed ourselves. I don't know why James said we could take care of you.' She was talking like they were poor when they were living in a five-bedroom house that had two TVs, several radios, and even a washer and dryer. There were carpets on the floors and all this stuff sitting around, plastic plants, little candy dishes, and whatnots that my mom could never have bought.

"At mealtime I was only allowed to eat one serving of vegetables while their kids had fried chicken or roast beef and all the helpings they wanted. They drank Kool-Aid and iced tea and I could only have water."

Rick shook his head and wrote something down. "Did you talk to your uncle about how she treated you?"

"No. Guess I knew he couldn't change it. Sometimes he'd get me to go out in the garage and work on cars with him. He'd even pay me a little money for helping out. I loved being with him and he taught me to always do my best at whatever I was doing, to take pride in my work."

"Did you tell your mom about your aunt?" Rick asked.

"Naw. Wouldn't have done no good. I'd just have ended up being called a no-good liar, like my father."

"Sounds like you were really alone no matter where you were."

"One time my mom came up for a visit. I remember I was very excited. The day she got there Aunt Ro laid out a beautiful spread with mashed potatoes, string beans, macaroni and cheese, fried chicken, biscuits and gravy. When she set a plate down in front of me that had a chicken wing on it I thought she'd made a mistake. I was afraid to even touch it. After we said grace and everybody started in, I just sat there.

"My mom said, 'Billy Junior, now you go on and eat. Don't be so rude. Your Aunt Ro's gone to a lot of trouble here, fixing all this good food.'

"I looked at her and then I looked at Aunt Ro. I can see her right now. She narrowed her eyes at me, then gave my mom a big smile. Then she looked back at me and said, 'Oh, stop being so shy, Billy Junior. Go on and eat.'

"I ate, but the food just sat in my stomach like a stone and I was really glad when I could leave the table."

I paused but Rick didn't say anything. I went on.

"Because Aunt Ro sent me to the store so often, it was easy for me to buy cigarettes. One day I was down in the basement and had just lit one up when Alyvia came downstairs and caught me. I tried to wave the smoke away but it was too late. She wanted a puff and at first I said, no way. But when she said she'd tell on me if I didn't let her, I gave in. She coughed a little with the first one, then wanted another one. And another one.

"In a way it felt good to put something over on Aunt Ro, but I should have known it wouldn't last. After the second or third time I'd let Alyvia smoke, Aunt Ro called me to come to the kitchen. I remember smelling the pot roast she was cooking for dinner. She was standing there with her hands on her hips and a big frown on her face. Uncle James stood beside her, looking like he'd rather be somewhere else. When I saw Alyvia sitting at the table crying, I knew she'd told on me.

"For three days I was only allowed to have bread and water, then Aunt Ro put me on the bus and sent me home two weeks early. That was the last time I stayed with Uncle James, which was okay with me. Being deprived of food at every meal made me feel like I was garbage. I swore to myself that when I was grown up I'd never treat anyone like that, and I'd always be able to eat whatever I wanted."

Rick looked at me and shook his head. "My God. That was downright cruel." He paused and looked at his watch. "I'm afraid we're about out of time for today," he said, "but we've made a good beginning here."

I got up and he shook my hand. As I left I thought about how this guy had really listened to me. And I had been honest, too. To the best of my ability. I felt cleaner, lighter, as I walked away.

◆   ◆   ◆

Our next meeting was two days later.

"We left off talking about your aunt and uncle," Rick said. "Today, let's talk about your dad. Where did he fit into all of this?"

I leaned forward, elbows on my knees, and looked at the floor. "He wasn't there. He never even sent me a birthday or Christmas card. That's all I knew. That, and the fact that my mother hated him. She always said he was no-good, a loser, and that I'd grow up to be just like him." I looked up at Rick. "But later I learned that he had a successful career in the Navy, and a nice home. I guess she always called him names because she hated him. I'm not sure why, but some of my relatives told me he was something of a ladies man.

"But I'll tell you that I was just a little kid when I understood that neither of my parents cared about me. My mother told me many times that I was nothing but a burden to her, and my father was completely absent. It was very clear to me that Aunt Lena and Uncle James were the only people who cared about me at all."

"I see," Rick said. "Did you get any support at school; say when you were in elementary school?"

"Well, I went to the first and second grades at a Catholic School. We had the kind of nuns who wore long black dresses and big wide hats that looked like wings. My mom was always saying if I studied hard maybe I wouldn't end up like my father. Anyway, I knew if I didn't do well in school, I'd get an ass beating.

"I didn't really like it. When I got into trouble for talking too much or giving a wrong answer, the nuns made me wear a dunce cap and sit in the front of the room, or they'd make me punch my fist into a brick wall ten times. I always felt like I got punished more than the others because I was one of the few black kids in the class and I wasn't Catholic. A couple of times I went to mass, trying to become part of the group, but it was nothing like our church. I didn't fit in."

"You were only there two years?" Rick asked. "Did you move away?"

"No," I said, shaking my head. "God, I wish we had. I got kicked out." That awful incident came back to me. This many years later I still felt the anger and the fear. "It all started one afternoon when me and my friend Joey rescued a little kitten from an old abandoned house across the street from where the nuns lived. When we stood by one of the windows we could just barely hear a weak meow. We looked inside and there was a gray kitten sitting on a pile of trash, crying. He was so little and he looked so scared. We decided to rescue that little thing, no matter what. I tried to push the window up but it wouldn't budge so we kept on looking till we found one that was cracked open. It was so high I couldn't move it, so we looked for something to stand on.

"It happened to be trash day and the nuns had put out cans for the garbage men to pick up. We took one of the smaller containers to the house, where I stood on it and shoved the window open. With Joey pushing from behind, I managed to get inside and pick up the kitten, who was still crying. He was so skinny I could feel his little ribs. His ears looked really big, maybe because he was so skinny."

As I spoke to Rick, I felt like I was back there, determined to rescue that helpless little thing. I was surprised at how clear it all was to me.

"Anyway, he was kind'a funny-looking but cute, you know. I could tell he was scared, and he never stopped meowing. I handed him through the window to

Joey and jumped down, and together we returned the trashcan. We ran to Joey's house where we poured some milk into a saucer and that little kitten lapped it up till his sides stuck out. Then he fell asleep on Joey's lap."

"How did you feel?" Rick asked.

"It was great! I was proud that we'd rescued that helpless little thing, and happy that Joey's mom said he could keep it. He turned into a pretty good-looking cat when he grew up. Those ears weren't so big after all."

"You rescued a skinny, scared, abandoned kitten with big ears."

I looked at him. "Yeah. That's right."

"Remind you of anybody?"

"The cat? Remind me of anybody? No."

"A skinny, scared, abandoned creature with big ears?"

I thought for a minute. "Me?" I said. "Me! He was just like me."

"And someone was there to rescue him. Who rescued you?"

I thought for a moment. "No one," I said. "I've always felt alone."

"Maybe there was more than one person who helped you through the years," he said.

I looked at a stack of books behind Rick. "How about your Aunt Lena?"

"Lena. Yes, Aunt Lena. I always knew she loved me," I said. "I couldn't say she rescued me, but I know she loved me."

"Anybody else? Maybe a teacher?"

"There was a nun. When I was in the first grade. She liked me. She was always good to me. And Mrs. Cradle, my teacher in a different school. She cared about me."

"Anybody else?"

I thought. "Coach Sticky. My high school basketball coach."

"So, it sounds like there were several people who came into your life who treated you well."

"Right. I guess so."

"So you weren't rescued all at once like that little kitten. You had little rescues along the way from Aunt Lena and your teachers.

I shook my head. "Damn! I never thought of it that way. I guess I am a little like that kitten." I smiled to myself. The puzzle pieces of my life started sliding into place.

"Well, Eugene, your ears don't look so big either," Rick said, laughing. "But let's get back to why you left the Catholic school."

"Oh yeah," I said. "Okay, well, one of the nuns must have seen us that day, and when it turned out that a trash container was missing, the head sister called me into her office the next morning and accused me of stealing it.

"I tried to tell her why we took it and that we put it back but she didn't have no ear to hear me. She just kept going on and on, saying I was lying and I was a thief for stealing from the church and God was gonna punish me for my sins. She said they didn't tolerate liars and thieves in their school and they were kicking me out and for me to wait in the hall while she called my mother."

Rick made some more notes.

"I sat in a chair just outside her door, my stomach twisted into knots, trying not to cry. It wasn't God I was afraid of. It was my mom. The hour I had to wait for her to get there seemed like ten. It was torture. When she finally came down the hall, she looked madder than I'd ever seen her. I was scared down to my bones. Without even looking at me, she went into the nun's office. A few minutes later she slammed the door open, grabbed my arm and dragged me down the steps to the sidewalk.

"I tried to tell her what happened, but she wouldn't listen either. After the first try, I knew it was hopeless. As we walked, she'd stop and jerk me around and get in my face. She was screaming, 'You little thief. You're just like your father!' She pinched me and slapped me. I tried to twist away but couldn't get loose. Then she'd drag me along for a few steps and we'd stop again. 'I had to leave my job for this, you little bastard. You know what that means, you little son of a bitch.' Whap, she hit me across the back of the head. Then she yelled, 'I'll bust your eyes and face open with my fists!' She pulled off a leather belt she was wearing and hit me across my back and butt over and over. Then she squeezed the back of my neck and said, 'I'll bust the eyes right out of your ugly face.'"

"Nobody on the street tried to intervene?"

"No way. When she was that mad nobody would mess with her. When we got home I ran to the closet without her even having to send me there. It was a relief to get locked in, all alone. I didn't even care that I didn't get any dinner."

I stopped talking. There was a long silence. Finally I said, "Today, I think what probably happened was that one of the containers was accidentally picked up by the trash men."

Rick shook his head. "Adults often don't listen to kids. Do you recall how you felt?"

"Damn right, I do. I felt humiliated. Worthless. Angry. Scared."

"Being ignored like that is painful."

"Ignored? I wish I'd just been ignored."

We both laughed and Rick said. "Did things like that happen to you often?"

I looked at him. "Well, sure. Especially where she was concerned."

"So the person who is supposed to protect you just turns you over to the wolves."

"That's right, in a way." I hesitated. "But she was one of the wolves."

"When you can't trust your parents, Tree, when you have no one to rely on, it can interfere with your ability to trust anybody. Even yourself."

I thought for a minute. It made sense that I didn't trust anybody. "I believe that."

"But you did have Aunt Lena. She was trustworthy. And that's really important. Hugely important. Without her, you might have become a very different man."

I smiled, once again feeling Aunt Lena beside me.

"Okay," Rick said. "So where did you go after you were expelled?"

"I went to Chestnut Street Elementary School. My teacher, Mrs. Cradle, was wonderful. My first day there she introduced me to the other children as Eugene, but told them to call me Billy. And, she said, because I'd just gotten out of the hospital for the second time, they couldn't play rough with me. I loved the special attention from her and felt like she coddled me, but the kids teased me and called me the teacher's pet. They said my name, Eugene, was a 'sissy' name. I'd never really gone by Eugene anyway, and after that I was sure I never would.

"That was when I started isolating myself from other kids by being 'a part of but not a part of' the group."

"What do you mean by that?" Rick asked.

"Oh, like I'd walk around the schoolyard as if I was counting the paces along the fence or checking out some bird in a tree. When I was with a group of kids I'd say something like, 'Oh, is that Malcolm over there? I've got to go see him.' Then when I got to Malcolm I'd find an excuse to go somewhere else. I was never comfortable with the other kids, always felt like I had to hide my real thoughts and feelings. If they knew who I really was, they'd never accept me."

"It's good you're aware of all that," said Rick. "You seem to have a pretty clear understanding of where you came up with some of the coping mechanisms you developed. When you started using them as a kid, it was because they worked. That's what we all do. But then, as we get older and those methods don't work anymore, we often keep on using them anyway because they're familiar. In a sense, it's doing the same thing over and over, expecting different results."

I nodded. "That's crazy. I know."

"Tell me about your mother."

Just thinking of her made me sweat. I wiped my face with my hands and took a deep breath. "Well, she was light-skinned, a handsome woman with a lot of energy. Her long hair was streaked with gray and she always dressed nice. She cared about what other people thought of her, but she had a fierce temper. When she was with other people she had a smile that looked warm and generous and she had lots of friends at church.

Until I was in junior high school, she was a nanny and cooked for the families of the Portsmouth Chief of Police and later, the editor of one of the big Norfolk newspapers. For years after she left those jobs, she was invited to attend the families' graduations, weddings, and funerals. She was even included in their wills.

"She always put in long hours at her day job, and at nights and on weekends she ran an illegal bootlegging business, selling liquor out of the house. The goal was to make money on the servicemen who wanted to get around the "Blue Laws" which prohibited the sale of alcohol after midnight and on Sundays. We lived near the naval shipyard, and when the bars closed it didn't take sailors long to find our house. Because my father was in the Navy, my mom was able to buy liquor on the Naval Base for less than it cost in the liquor stores, and sell it for a profit.

"I started pouring drinks for the customers when I was nine or ten, and within a couple of years I was stealing whiskey out of the bottles regularly, and replacing it with water. That made me popular with my friends, and my mom never seemed to notice.

"You started drinking pretty early, then."

"Yeah, I guess I did. Alcohol was always around. Easy to get. By the time I was thirteen or fourteen, I was drinking alcoholically."

"Tell me more about that."

"Well, drinking was just a part of growing up. When I drank, I felt like I fit in. For once, I was a part of the crowd. It was the only time I felt like I was normal. And bootlegging was never a moral problem to anyone I knew. I grew up in a world of hypocrisy—things were never what they seemed. My mom's customers, who constantly got drunk and cheated on their husbands and wives, didn't see anything wrong with doing that. People who stole and robbed for a living were sitting on the front row at church every Sunday. They justified their illegal 'work' by saying they couldn't earn enough from one job to get by, but I don't think that was really the case. If they had put as much energy into their regular jobs as they did into the illegal ones, they might have come out okay."

"Hmmm," Rick said. "Drinking and stealing were just normal parts of everyday life."

"Right. Another way people got money was gambling. There was always a Tunk game going on somewhere."

"Tunk game?" Rick said.

"It's a card game. The way it worked was that whoever was holding the game in their home sold food and liquor to the others and also collected a percentage of the pot. The bets ranged from fifty cents to five or ten dollars a hand. The only catch was that to be a part of the group, you had to agree to play when other people held games, and help them out in a pinch."

"That's a good idea," Rick said. "I could see that helping out."

"Oh, it did. It did."

"Did you have any other family around?"

"Not in town. But during the summers, when she was having trouble making ends meet, my mom sent me to visit relatives or friends of hers who lived out in the country. Sometimes I stayed with her younger sisters, Aunt Peggy and Aunt Piggy, over in Accomack.

When I was with them, I read a lot. Books were an easy way to escape from the world. Of all my relatives, their home was the best place to stay because they gave me a little room of my own where I could disappear with a book for as long as I wanted. They gave me lots of hugs and lots of cookies, and I loved being there. They lived back in the country where people didn't have street addresses; you're known for where the oak tree fronts the road and you're five houses to the right or ten houses behind it. Everybody knew everybody else, and they were all very friendly."

"Different from the city life, I guess."

"Yeah, right, man. In some ways, anyhow. But my aunts were bootleggers, like my mom. Aunt Peggy was the businesswoman, bringing people into their place, cleaning up the tables and handling the money. Aunt Piggy was, for lack of a better description, a happy drunken lady who had some mental problems and always made a mess of everything she tried to do. She'd pass out from drinking, and she could be extremely funny or very sad. She'd put her finger in her mouth in a childlike way, look at you out of the corner of her eye, and then burst into laughter. The family was very protective of her.

"Then for a couple of summers I stayed with my Aunt Leevy, who was really just a friend of my mom's. She and her husband, Billy, lived about fifteen miles away in Fentress, where the water always smelled like rotten eggs. They made moonshine and sold it in the downstairs of their home, just like my mom and aunts did. Aunt Leevy let me earn a few tips sometimes, serving drinks to customers. Once in a while she'd even let me have some beer.

"But I didn't fit in with the kids out there. The boys called me 'city kid,' and when they found a snake, they'd come over and call me outside, then chase me with it or throw it at me. When I ran they called me a 'scaredy cat.' I remember thinking I was too old to cry about somebody calling me names. But the snakes scared the shit out of me. Still do."

Rick laughed. "I don't like them either, and nobody ever threw one at me!"

I laughed with him.

"But at least you had exposure to places other than the city. To different kinds of families."

"You're right, Rick. I learned that everybody's home life wasn't like mine."

Life Painted by Number

◆

1998

When we talked about our addictions in group therapy, some of the men said they grew frustrated quickly when they weren't able to solve their problems right away. "Patience, you have to learn patience," the counselors told us over and over. "You have to be able to delay gratification. It took a long time for you to get to the place you're in, and it'll take a while to get out." They had lots of ideas about how we could practice patience, and the one that appealed to me was to get a hobby.

When I was a kid I used to like the paint-by-number pictures, so I bought one of the Last Supper down in the hospital gift shop. When I opened the box and saw all those little tiny areas I'd have to paint, I thought maybe I should have gotten something simpler. Then I reminded myself that I was in the process of taking action to achieve a goal I'd set for myself. I needed to take one step at a time. I decided to work on it every day for thirty minutes before lunch, and maybe thirty minutes before dinner.

First I painted all the spots marked with the number 1, blue. When I started putting white on the number 2's, my hand accidentally smeared it over the blue paint. When I tried using the brush without resting my hand on the canvas, I couldn't control the brush.

To get some new ideas, I checked out library books on painting. One of them suggested picking a certain area to work on and going from left to right to prevent smudging. I also started using a "level stick" to steady my hand and a magnifying glass to see the smallest areas. One of the men in our group was something of an artist, and when I asked for his help, he showed me how to pick out brushes and cut the edges to make fine points for the smallest sections.

As my painting progressed, I got more interested in it. The half-hour before lunch and dinner expanded to include a half-hour after lunch and dinner. Gradually, I added my break times plus an hour or two before I went to sleep. The longer I worked at it, the better I got. I even changed some of the colors to bring out areas I wanted to emphasize.

When I finished, what I saw was a program of recovery. At first I had followed directions. Then I got more information and asked for help. Finally, I took action. In the beginning I made mistakes, but I didn't give up.

In my painting there were rough areas and smooth ones; some colors were bright and others dark. The more I put into my project, the better results I got.

Follow directions. Get information. Ask for help. Take action.

◆   ◆   ◆

After several more sessions I had no hesitation about talking with Rick; I even looked forward to it. By the time I'd seen him five or six times, it was like visiting an old friend.

"How's it going?" he asked one afternoon.

"Good," I said. "I've been remembering things I haven't thought of in years."

"That happens sometimes," he said. "Any of them related to your mother?"

"How did you know?"

He smiled at me. "Just a lucky guess. We'd talked a while back about your staying with her sisters in the summers. But what was it like to live with her?"

I sighed. "Well, we didn't really get along. When I was around she was almost always short-tempered; it was her way or the highway. She was always telling me what to do and I don't think I ever had a real give-and-take conversation with her. Our talks usually went something like this: 'Now, you listen to me, you little bastard. If that teacher calls me one more time about your grades or the way you been cuttin' up, I'll bust your eyes and face open with my fists.'"

"That's quite a threat!" Rick said. "Did she ever do that?"

"Well, she never hit me in the face but she sure hit me everywhere else."

"Was she ever affectionate?"

I looked at a stack of books on the floor by Rick's desk. The top one must have had fifty post-it notes sticking out of the pages. *Affectionate,* I thought. *Was she ever affectionate?*

"Well, she hugged me once in a while, but just when we were with other people. The only time she seemed to even want to be in the same room with me was when she had friends over from the church. Then she'd say something like, 'Ain't my Billy Junior tall and handsome?' And I'd feel so good. But as soon as her friends left, she'd turn on me. 'Why you acting like a fool in front of the church sisters?' she'd say. Or, 'You just as stupid as your no-good father.'"

"Can you remember a time when you felt like she was a good mother?" Rick asked.

I looked out the window and thought hard. Finally, I said, "Once in a while she'd give me money to go to the store and get some cookies or chocolate ice cream. Then we'd sit at the kitchen table and eat it. But always in silence. We never just talked or played games or anything like that. There was always something she had to be doing, or something I had to be doing, or something I wasn't doing that I should have been doing. I liked it better when I was at home alone."

"What did you do when your mom was at home with you?" Rick asked.

"Leave the house, or more often, stay in my room. That is, unless she was in her bedroom. There was a door connecting our rooms and I was forbidden to go into hers without permission. At night, I often heard men in there, talking and laughing, sometimes yelling and moaning. Sometimes there were fights—lots of screaming and crashing around."

"How did you react to that?" Rick asked.

"I was scared. Sometimes I pulled my pillow over my head. Or I hid in the closet where I kept a pillow crammed in the back to use when she sent me in there to punish me. And I had a little flashlight for some light if I got scared. When it finally got quiet I'd make pictures in my head of how other people lived and imagine having the perfect family, like those old TV shows in the 1950's, *Leave it to Beaver* and *Father Knows Best*. I wanted to live with a mother and father who loved me. Or I'd come up with a story where I was the hero. Sometimes it seems to me that I spent more time in my closet than I did in my bedroom."

"What was your mom's life like when she was growing up?"

It took me a minute to think. "She never talked about it," I said, looking up at him. "I know she was the oldest of three girls and they were from somewhere down south, Alabama, I think. They lived way out in the country and had no running water; they used a generator for electricity. Now, I remember that once I went down to Alabama with her, to her dad's funeral. Somewhere way out in the country." I leaned back, remembering that time so long ago.

"His house was just a shack. Didn't look like it had ever been painted. It sat in a clearing along a dirt road by a railroad track, with five or six other cabins just like it. It looked to me like they could have been slave quarters. A bare light bulb hung from the ceiling in the main room, but they also had oil lamps and candles throughout the house because the generator didn't work all the time."

I hadn't thought of those details in years.

"He cooked on a potbellied wood stove and outside, there was a hand pump for water. He even had an outhouse."

"My God. They were really poor," Rick said.

"When we first got there, the house was full of these great big people. The women were dressed in the same kinds of flowery dresses Aunt Peggy and Aunt Piggy always wore, and they all looked rough. But they seemed kindhearted and were really glad to see my mom.

"Before we left, my mom learned her dad had left her something that was very special to him. It was a parchment, all rolled up in a box. I remember being disappointed that it wasn't a lot of money, but I guess that's all he had. He was one of the original members of the first groups of black Masons in that area, and he'd told everybody that the paper had been signed by the original founders of the organization in Alabama. He'd left my mom the most precious thing he owned."

"He must have loved her," Rick said.

"Yeah, I guess he did," I said.

Rick made another note. "Sounds like your mother probably didn't have it very easy as a kid." He paused. "You know, Eugene," he said, "sometimes it helps to look at your parents as people, instead of just as your parents. In spite of everything, it sounds like your mom always provided you with food and shelter. Maybe that's the best she could do."

I looked down at the floor. I'd never considered that. "Well, maybe."

"It could be that for your mom, living in the city was better than where she grew up."

I'd never thought about it that way. But it made sense. "Yeah," I said. "Maybe so. But you know, I needed her to show me that she loved me, give me a hug once in a while."

"Do you think it's possible that she didn't know how to show love? Maybe her family didn't show any love to her when she was a child." Rick paused, but I didn't say anything. "At least she never abandoned you."

"I guess you're right. She never did. She even came to see me in jail after I'd told her not to."

"So, maybe she showed you she cared in the only way she knew how." He paused and shifted in his seat. "Some kids find supportive adults at church. Did you and your mom go to church?"

"Oh, sure. Church. My mom was one of the elders and a member of the pastor's board. She also acted as a nurse during services. She'd put smelling salts to people's noses when they fainted, or hold people so that they wouldn't hurt themselves when they were shouting or full of the spirit. It seemed to me that she was very important.

"When I was about nine, she made me sign up to be a Junior Usher. I hated it because I had to get all dressed up—even wore white gloves—and I had to stand in the middle of the aisle in one certain spot for the entire service. When people needed fans or prayer books I went and got them, but the rest of the time I just stood there. I didn't like it, but I must admit it did give me a sense of importance. About that time my mom decided I should be a Cub Scout and she volunteered to be the den mother."

Rick looked up, surprise on his face. "Your mom was a den mother?"

"Yep, she was." I nodded and smiled, remembering. "And I was really proud to have her in charge. It was all very organized and every month we'd work on a new merit badge. She'd look in the book and pick one out for me. Of course, when it wasn't perfect I got a smack or a pinch, and she'd say, 'You just too damn stupid. You worse than your father.' I did my best, but the knots I made never looked as good as hers, and I couldn't remember which footprints went with which animal no matter how hard I tried. In the end, she just finished most of my projects for me. That year I got more merit badges than anybody else and was crowned 'King of the Scouts' at church. I was so proud."

"So, at least some of the time your mom tried to do the right thing."

"Well," I said, "sometimes she did. You're right. Sometimes she did. And we never went hungry. I always had clothes, usually hand-me-downs she brought home from work." I laughed. "'Course all my friends would be dressed in jeans and All Star tennis shoes with pullover T-shirts, and here I'd come along wearing the 'too short' khaki pants low on my hips which made the seat hang down around my knees. And I had these expensive brown penny loafers and button-down shirts. I was something to see."

Rick laughed and I found myself joining in. It felt good to be able to laugh at something that had only caused me pain until now. "But once in a while I got something new. I remember it was a big deal for me one Easter when she bought me a suit. I was so excited to have new clothes like the other boys. It was the first time I remember feeling like I really looked good. While the ladies set up our pot-luck dinner after church, I ran to the merry-go-round on the side of the church-yard. Three other kids were already on it, spinning real fast and they called for me to get on. I tried to grab onto the metal bar but I slipped and tore a hole in the knee of my new pants. I was upset about ruining the pants, but far more than that, I was afraid of what my mom would do when she saw them.

"I sat with my friends to eat Easter dinner so I could put off having to face her, but I couldn't even eat the fried chicken, my favorite." As I talked, the feelings of fear and dread filled me. I felt like I was nine years old again, helpless, at the mercy of the one person in the world who was supposed to love me. Tears filled my eyes. I cleared my throat.

Rick silently handed me a box of tissues.

"When we got home and she saw what I'd done, she said, 'Strip off them clothes you just ruined. I ain't gonna hurt that suit I just paid for, but I'm sure as hell gonna beat your ass, you little bastard.'" My voice cracked and I had to stop talking. I cleared my throat again and wiped my face. "I pulled off the jacket and shirt, crying, knowing there was nothing I could do to stop her. 'Faster, you little son of a bitch!' she said. 'Get them pants off!' When I hesitated, she hit me and said, 'Faster, faster.'"

Embarrassed, I glanced up at Rick, then down at the floor, wiping the wetness from my face. It was a minute before I could continue.

"When I was standing in front of her, naked, she came at me with the buckle end of a leather belt. I screamed and cried, but that just made her madder and she hit me harder. I'll never forget that beating."

"My God, Eugene. You've survived some awful things," Rick said. "Really awful."

I looked back at him as tears rolled down my cheeks.

Lucius or Lucifer?

◆

1998

Along with going to therapy, I attended every AA meeting that was brought into the domiciliary by alcoholics living in the community. One night, when the topic was about changing, a man wearing an orange shirt, yellow tie, green pants, and a plaid jacket raised his hand. He said when he first came into the program he wore dark baggy clothes and tried to look intimidating, but the old timers knew he was dressing to cover up his fear. While he wanted to be a part of the program, he thought if people got to know him they wouldn't want anything to do with him. When he started dressing differently, people saw him as friendlier, and he actually became friendlier.

I began to realize that there were many ways of keeping people at a distance. Although I'd always been a neat dresser, I wondered what I might be doing to hide. I thought about how when I was with other people, I was good at acting like I was a part of the group, but I never felt a part of it. I'd been holding back like I'd done in the schoolyard as a kid; the same behavior I'd used to my advantage in the penitentiary. But that skill was now a liability—a way I'd been keeping myself separate from others, never letting them get to know me. I started trying to change that, and slowly I made progress. I made sure I got to meetings early to help set up, and stayed late to clean up. Although it felt awkward at first, I started getting to know people.

One night Lady G., the Night Director of our Domiciliary (Dom), told me something I've never forgotten. She said, "Don't let your friends pick you, Eugene. You pick your friends." That made good sense to me. I started deciding who I wanted to be with instead of allowing others to choose me. I learned to set boundaries, as Rick would say, and stopped putting myself in uncomfortable positions. If I was asked to go somewhere I didn't want to go, or with someone I didn't feel comfortable with, I could say, 'No thanks.' Then, when I was with people I liked, I could really be myself and feel a part of the group.

I also decided to start going by my real name, Eugene. Ever since the kids had teased me about it in the second grade, I'd never wanted to be called Eugene. I'd always thought Billy sounded more macho. But now, I said to myself, if Eugene is really my name, and I truly want to stop hiding and let people know who I am, maybe I should use it. One thing for sure, "Billy" is not the man I wanted to be.

I looked up the name Eugene and learned that it comes from the Greek and means "The Most Trusted," or "Trusted Friend." I even heard that Jesus' disciple who took Judas' place was named Eugene.

◆   ◆   ◆

Rick was running late for our next meeting, so I had to wait fifteen minutes. I was starting to feel irritated, thinking I wouldn't have my full hour with him—so different from the way I'd felt in other treatment programs. While I waited, I thought about where we'd left off last time, talking about the worst beating my mom had ever given me. For the first time, I wondered if she'd ever been beaten as a child. I decided she probably had.

When Rick got there, he apologized for the delay, then looked at his notes and asked, "Was it always just you and your mother? Did she ever marry again?"

I took a deep breath. "Oh yeah. She sure did. I was eight, I think, when she met Lucius Estes. He was one of the sailors who came to our house to buy bootleg liquor. My mom always had lots of boyfriends so I didn't pay much attention to him, then all of a sudden he was living with us. From the beginning, without ever saying a word, Lucius made it clear that he didn't want me around. I didn't know anything about them getting married, but I heard them tell other people that they had. Lucius was attracted to my mom and I think she was interested in his Navy retirement check.

"We moved into a big old two-story colonial style house near the Fourth Street gate of the Naval Station. The sounds from the shipyard were always in the background, big machinery clanging, whistles going off, and people talking and yelling.

"We were one of five black families living in the middle of a white neighborhood, and six of us boys became close friends. We went everywhere together because there was safety in numbers. You never knew when white people might drive through the streets yelling, 'Porch monkeys!' and 'Nigger go home,' while they waved rebel flags. They'd blow their car horns and sometimes threw eggs or fruit at us. It was never really safe—none of us kids were ever allowed to go to the store alone."

"Tell me about Lucius," Rick said.

I looked down and shook my head. "He was short and barrel-chested and smelled like sweat and gin, even in the mornings before he started drinking. His eyes were always red, and they reminded me of the red eyes I'd seen in pictures of the devil. At first I tried to find ways to make him like me. I'd get his bedroom slippers or newspaper or take him a beer. But it didn't work.

As I looked up at Rick, a sour old memory came back. "One winter afternoon, a few months after he moved in, I had my first real run-in with him. A couple of friends had walked home from school with me, and when we got in front of my house, my buddy Arno, who was much bigger than me, gave me a shove. He was just teasing, and said, 'Go on home, mama's boy.' We threw out a few punches like we were going to fight, and Lucius stepped out from the porch and yelled, 'Hey, what's going on? Kick his ass, Billy Junior. Come on! Come on here now!' He started walking our way, yelling, 'Don't be such a sissy, Billy Junior. Kick that little bastard's ass.'

"I said, 'But, Lucius.'

"By this time he was standing over us, yelling, holding a drink in his hand. 'You hear me boy? I ain't raisin' no sissy. Now, you little bastard! Now! If you don't kick his ass, I'm gonna kick your ass.' We all just stood there staring at him.

"I hit Arno in the stomach and on his shoulder and then, with almost no effort at all, he tripped me and shoved me backwards, down to the ground. Then they left.

"Lucius snatched me up by the front of my jacket and pulled me up to his drunken face. He was drooling and spitting and smelled like alcohol and cigarettes. 'You gotta learn to defend yourself and stop actin' like a punk,' he said. 'You got to be tough, not soft. You don't get nothing in this world lessen you take it. You always got to be a man. Take what you want. Fight any asshole who gets in your way.'"

"Tough guy," Rick said. "Now you were living with two abusive adults."

"You got that right," I said.

"Did you have any brothers or sisters?"

"My half-sister, Ivy, was born a few months after that run-in, and that's when I gave up trying to please Lucius. Ivy was all he and my mom cared about. He took care of Ivy and ran my mom's bootlegging business while she worked at Hagwood's Dry Cleaners. I remember being surprised at how gentle he could be with a baby.

"When Lucius drank he was cruel, and he drank a lot. He and my mom had huge fights that sometimes involved knives and a lot of blood. When I heard them starting up, I ran into my room, or into the closet to hide. I'd listen to them yelling and cursing at each other while dishes crashed and bodies thudded against the walls or furniture. One time I got in between them and yelled at him to stop hurting my mom, but she slapped me and screamed at me to go to my room. I never tried that again.

"Lucius' temper was well known, and when he came home after drinking at some other bootlegger's place, all the sailors at our house left. When my mom was mad at him, she'd tell me his name meant Lucifer, and Lucifer was the Devil."

"You mentioned that your mother welcomed the financial security Lucius brought with him. Do you think she cared about him other than that?"

"I don't know. Maybe at first. If she did, it didn't last long. I don't remember him ever putting his arm around her, or her ever giving him a kiss."

"Did they ever go out together? Have friends over?"

I laughed. "You kidding me? They was running a bootlegging house. It was full of people all the time. I guess you could call some of 'em friends, but there was always a lot of people around. Lucius would be there during the day, but when my mom was home he'd go out driving around and visiting other bootleggers. He had this blue '59 Buick he was so proud of—he loved racing the engine.

"When he pulled up out front and started revving the motor, 'Rhumm, rhummmm, rhummmm,' it was a very bad sign. A dark, scary feeling always came over me then. I knew he'd been drinking and what was coming next.

"I could never decide which of Lucius' moods was worse. When he was in a pleasant drunken mood, he might try to play with me, like maybe teach me to fight. But whatever we did, I always ended up getting hurt. If we didn't play games, he made fun of me or I had to listen to him brag about what a tough guy he was in the Navy.

"When he was on an angry drunk he called me names and told me how worthless I was, that I was not his kid and was just a freeloader, like my no-good father. When he started in on me, my mother never said a word. Eventually, I just went to the closet on my own as soon as I heard him gunning the car's engine."

"Was it all bad? Was Lucius ever anything but unkind?"

I had to think. "Well, a few times he took me along when he went to visit other bootleggers or his girlfriends, and then he was almost friendly. But when my mom was with us, he was always critical."

"Is Lucius still around?"

"No. He died when I was thirteen. I came home from school one afternoon and found my mom there with lots of other people from the church. She said he had collapsed at one of the other bootlegger's houses and they took him to the hospital, but it was too late. I never saw her shed a tear over him. After that day I don't remember her ever mentioning him again. I think she was more relieved than anything else. She said she'd had enough. She never married again."

A Letter to My Father

✦

1998

During a session the following week, Rick asked, "How did you get along after Lucius died? Did he leave your mom any money?"

"No way. He drank it all up. I guess she got some allotment for Ivy, but she still had to work at the laundry and pick up extra jobs on the weekends. Before long, she and Ivy and I moved to a renovated garage that was just one big room. In one corner there was a little bathroom that always smelled like pee, and next to that was a small kitchen sink with couple of cabinets under it, and a small stove.

"We had no Christmas tree that year and there was only one gift, a Barbie Doll for Ivy. The men who came to buy liquor from my mom felt sorry for me and started giving me money, which made me feel a little better. But after Ivy broke the head off her Barbie Doll, she went crying to every man who came in, and with tears streaming down her cheeks, told them her sad tale. They said I had to split my money with her, which I didn't like at all. I always wondered if she broke that doll on purpose."

Rick laughed.

"How about your dad? Had you met him by this time?"

"No. I always thought he was far away in the Navy, but then I got a surprise. The first day after school let out for that next summer, that was after Lucius died, my mom told me I couldn't go visit Aunt Leevy because she didn't have money for the bus fare. Instead I was going to stay with my father. Turned out he'd been living in town for a long time, only ten or twelve blocks away. That was news to me.

"Why do you think she hadn't told you?"

"I'm not sure." I hesitated. "You know, she hated him so much. Maybe she thought I'd try to find him or something. And find out that all those ugly things she'd always said about him weren't true. I don't know."

"Must have been a real shock."

"Yeah. It was. She told me he sure didn't want to have to take me and he tried to say they didn't have room, 'but that's tough shit,' she said. 'Now he's got his own little family, he don't want nothing to do with us. But he ain't getting off that easy.' She said she'd promised herself she'd never ask my pop for help, but I was such a burden she didn't have a choice. She said I had to go the next day, right after she got off work.

"All I'd ever heard about my father was that he was a terrible person and I'd never wanted anything to do with him. In the only photo I'd ever seen of him, he was wearing a sailor uniform and a white cap and he looked confident and successful. In the background was the ship he served on with the words "USS Independence" handwritten across the bottom. I used to stare at that picture and wonder if I'd look like him when I grew up.

"It scared me to think of living with this man who was supposed to be so awful, such a "no-good," who my mom said had put beer in my baby bottle to shut up my crying. He'd never been a father to me.

"I wondered what he would think of me. If he'd like me. I was so skinny and ugly I knew there was no way he could be proud of me. But maybe he would be. Maybe he'd even love me. I knew that was too much to hope for. But I hoped for it anyway.

I stopped talking. I felt numb. Remembering.

"Did you go?" Rick asked.

I looked up at him.

"To your dad's, I mean."

"Ohhhh, yeah. I went." I heard the bitterness in my own voice. "When my mom came home from work the next afternoon she was yelling at me to hurry up before she even got to the door. She had borrowed a car and said she had things to do with Ivy.

"When we pulled up at my father's place I couldn't believe what I saw. The yard was neatly trimmed and there were flowers of all colors along the front. The house was a clean pink and white and there was a big pink and white Oldsmobile in the driveway. I stared at it as my mom said, 'Get the hell out the car. Go on! Get out! I ain't got all day.'

"I didn't move. 'Get out Billy,' she said. 'This is the place. Get out the fucking car and go on in.'

"I was so scared I just sat there, frozen. 'If you don't get the hell out I'll bust your eyes and face open with my fists,' she said.

"I held on tight to my brown paper bag of clothes and got out. The tires screeched as the car pulled away from the curb. My mom never looked back, but

Ivy smiled at me and waved. I walked up to the door feeling more alone than I'd ever felt in my life. What if I was at the wrong house? What if he'd changed his mind and wouldn't let me stay there? I knew he didn't want me. I took a deep breath and tried to look brave. I walked up to the door and knocked. A lady opened it and smiled at me.

"'You must be Billy Junior,' she said. 'Come on in here, child. Oh, my, you look just like your father. I'm Cleo, your daddy's wife.' Then she put her hand on my shoulder and said, 'Come on in this way. He's waiting for you in the den. Don't be afraid.'

"As we walked down the hall I could feel my heart pounding in my chest. And there he was. My father was sitting at his desk. He was slender with a gray/black mustache and his wavy gray hair was parted down the middle. He wore a tan suit with a dark blue tie. He had such an air of authority that I knew I had to obey him without question. He stood up and put out his hand. I shifted the paper bag to my left arm and reached out to him. When we shook he put his left hand around the back of my neck, the way you would with a good friend, and I felt hopeful for the first time.

"He said, 'I've been looking forward to spending some time with you, Billy Junior.' I was so nervous I couldn't even talk. I just nodded. He asked if my mom told me he'd been sending money for me every month and I mumbled something that I hoped sounded like yes, but I didn't know anything about any money. He sat back down and told Mama Cleo to show me the bedroom I'd be sharing with her son, Calvin.

"'Come on, Honey,' she said, putting her hand on my shoulder and steering me further down the hall. She showed me the bed I'd be sleeping in and said, 'My boy Calvin is at the college right now, but he'll be home before too long. In the meantime,' she said, pointing to the bottom dresser drawer, 'you can just put your stuff in that drawer there. He emptied it out for you. And there are some magazines on the bedside table that you can read till suppertime.'

"I was worried that Calvin might not want me there, but it turned out that wasn't the case. When he got home I heard him call out, 'Mama, where's my little brother?' then I heard his footsteps sounding in the hall. I put down the magazine I was reading and scrambled to my feet. He came in smiling and shook my hand. 'Welcome, Billy Junior,' he said. 'Looks like we're gonna be roommates for a while.'"

"So how did it work out at your dad's?" Rick asked.

"Well, with few exceptions, the time I spent 'getting to know' my father was at the dinner table. We ate every night at six sharp, and if you weren't there right on time you'd better have a good reason. When we sat down to eat the second night, Pop said, 'What did you do today, Billy Junior? Did you help Cleo around the house?'

"I hadn't even thought of offering to help. I broke out in a cold sweat. I said, 'No, sir. I went to the park this morning and read books in my room all afternoon.'

"'Well,' he said, 'first off, you need to know that my wife is not your maid. You need to carry your share of the load around here. We all carry our fair share.' I was humiliated.

"Then he wanted to know what I'd been reading. When I told him it was comic books, he said that kind of trash wasn't allowed in his house, and that I had to throw them all out. He thought it was awful my mom let me read them.

"By that time I had no appetite, but he insisted it was rude not to eat the food Mama Cleo had cooked. So I picked up my fork and ate, but I couldn't taste a thing. When I looked over at Mama Cleo, she winked at me. Later while I dried the dishes, she told me not to worry, that his bark was worse than his bite. She even said he loved me. I wanted so much to believe her.

"Every night at dinner Pop lectured me about how hard he'd had it in his day, and every night my appetite went right out the window. He'd say, 'You have to learn to support yourself. You can't always sit back and let everybody else do all the work. You have to pull your own weight.'

"After he'd chastised me for something I'd done, Mama Cleo would bring me a cookie or come up with ways to help me get out of trouble. Sometimes I felt she was more of a mother to me than my own mother was. At least she was kinder to me."

Rick asked, "Did it get any better as the summer went on?"

"Well, I guess I got used to living there. I got along fine with Calvin and Mama Cleo. They made me feel at home. But living in a well-kept neighborhood was a new experience and I was surprised that everyone knew each other. I didn't make friends with the kids who lived nearby because somehow they all seemed to know I was my father's bastard child—that I wasn't as good as they were. Every time I started playing with the girl who lived next door, her mother called her to come in within just a few minutes. After the first several times it was clear that she didn't want me around. Again, I felt like an outcast. I didn't fit in."

"Did you spend any time with your dad that you enjoyed?"

"Well, two or three times he took me down to the Elk's Lodge with him, where he was the Secretary, Treasurer, and bartender. He sat me on a bar stool and gave me a soda, and when the other men and women asked about me he'd say, 'This is my son, Billy Junior.' The ladies would smile and say, 'You're just as handsome as your daddy,' and the men would ask, 'How many girlfriends you got?' But when we went home, my father was always tough with me. He'd emphasize spiritual lessons and moral values, but I felt like he was just criticizing me.

"He and my mom both turned into different people when others weren't around. There was such a difference between their homes, and between my mother and Mama Cleo, that it was hard for me to figure out where I stood. Seemed to me I didn't belong anywhere at all."

"I can see why."

"When the summer was over I was glad to get back to my mom's where there weren't so many rules. By that time she and Ivy had moved to an apartment in the projects."

"That was just before you started high school?"

"Yeah. That's right."

"What were you like as a teenager?" Rick asked. "When did you really start drinking?"

"Well, like I said, I was stealing my mom's liquor when I was nine or ten I guess, and drinking pretty steady by the time I was thirteen. At night I'd meet my friends for a few beers before we went down to the teen dance hall. But before I left home I'd have already finished off a six-pack of beer or a bottle of wine—it took that to work up the courage to go. We were already drunk by the time we got to the hall, so it didn't matter that alcohol wasn't allowed. And being drunk, I didn't keep my eye on the clock to be sure I got home on time, so sometimes my mom came looking for me, yelling her head off.

"'Goddamn you! What did I tell you?' Whap, she'd hit me in the back of the head in front of my friends. 'You coming home with me right now,' she'd say, kicking and hitting wherever she could reach me. When she couldn't find me, she locked me out of the house, so I often stayed with one of the other boys.

"I have to say she did her best to control me, and I think in her eyes she was being a good mother. The more she tried to hold me back, the harder I fought it. To me it was simple, I just wanted to stay out with my friends whose curfews were later than mine. I'd often just be in the front yard or standing down the street with some of my buddies. She knew all the boys I hung out with and it seemed to me that she could see we weren't doing anything wrong."

"Okay now," Rick said, leaning forward. "You said your mother died, right?"

"Yeah. She died last summer."

"Did you ever make any amends to her while she was alive?"

"No. She lived up in Virginia and she'd been out of her head with Alzheimer's for a few years."

"What would you think about writing her a letter? She may not be here anymore, but you can still make some amends."

"I guess I could do that," I said. "I guess so."

"Good, that's good. And how about your dad? He's still alive, isn't he?"

"That's right."

"Have you been in touch with him lately?"

"No."

"Think you might want to contact him and let him know where you are?"

Humiliation and anger filled me, just thinking of him. He'd deserted me. I wanted to forget he'd ever existed. "He don't care about me," I said, looking at the floor and shaking my head. "And I don't care about him."

"I know he wasn't around when you were a little kid, Tree. But in a way he was there—in a manner of speaking. Think of it as his shadow being there. You always had a father."

I didn't say anything.

"Every child has feelings about his parents, even when they don't know where they are. Or even who they are. What I'm saying is that his absence didn't just leave an empty space. That space was full of feelings."

"Well, those feelings aren't good ones."

"That may be true. For now. But things can change. You can change. I want you to consider writing to him."

"When I write, he never writes back. I wait to hear from him, and when I get no answer, I feel awful. Sometimes Mama Cleo has answered my letters, but I know I'm a big disappointment."

"Well now, put yourself in your dad's place for a minute," Rick said. "He has a son who's an addict, who's been to prison three times and lived on the streets for years. I'm sure that's not what he wanted for you. Might not hurt to just write him and tell him that you're still alive."

My whole body tensed. "Well, I don't know," I said, glancing at Rick. "Then I'll have to feel his disappointment in me again, or I'll be hoping he'll write back and end up waiting for a letter that never comes. Or I'll get a letter from Mama Cleo instead of him. I don't want no more of that."

"You don't have to tell him where you are, you know. That way you won't have to expect a letter. Just send it without a return address. That way he can't write back, but you'll have done your part to be a responsible son. He'll want to know that you're alive and in a safe place. You owe him that respect."

"Well, I'll think about it. Maybe I will." I reminded myself that I needed to take action and follow suggestions.

That night I wrote both letters. I told my mom I was sorry I hadn't been able to change my life while she was still alive, and that I regretted a lot of things I'd done. I was especially sorry that I wasn't around to help her at the end of her life, even though she wouldn't have known who I was.

The one to my father was short. It said, "Pop, I just want to let you know that I'm in a safe place and I'm doing okay, Billy Junior."

One of the Boys

✦

1998

In group therapy we talked about the power of the family, how our early lives helped shape the people we'd become, and that as bad as it may have been, our parents probably did the best they could. We studied our thinking patterns and learned how to reason a problem all the way through to its resolution. We talked a lot about the Twelve Steps. I'd been introduced to them so many times in treatment centers that I knew what I needed to do. Like before, I excelled in expressing myself, but this time I did my best to do it honestly and to follow Rick's suggestions to take some action. And that made all the difference. After talking to him honestly, I felt more hopeful and more responsible, like I was actually in the process of becoming the man I wanted to be.

The group therapy counselor said we needed to understand why we'd chosen to use drugs and alcohol. "Remember situations you were in when you drank," he'd say. "Think about it. How were you feeling? What was going on before? Afterwards? Did you try not to drink?"

We talked about the details, what kind of environments we were living in, our jobs, earnings, friends, family, everything. In group therapy we talked about our childhoods and the counselor pushed us to be honest about our thoughts and feelings. Especially our fears.

He warned us, "Some of you will be likely to say what you think you're supposed to say, but that won't help you get sober. You have to be honest, get to the bottom of things." To keep us focused on the truth he taught us to ask each other during the meetings, "Are you speaking from the heart, or off the top?"

◆   ◆   ◆

"Okay," Rick said, as we sat down at one of our later sessions. "Last time we left off talking about when you moved. Just before you started high school, I think. Let's start there."

"Okay. Let's see. My mom got a better paying job, bought herself a car and we moved to the public housing apartments, right across from the school I was going to attend. But it was not a good place to live. Because of the poverty, drug use and criminal element in the neighborhood, within a few years it grew to be such a dangerous area that it was called 'Little Vietnam.' Guns, alcohol and drugs were everywhere.

"The layout of the projects had lots of places to run in and out of, making it easy to hide. Everybody there sold something out of their apartments, food, drinks, ice cream, and all kinds of dope. Some of the older people 'held' items, like drugs, and kept them safe till the owner needed them. For a price, of course. Since gunshots were frequent, there was an unwritten rule that any children who were outside when shots were heard would be brought into the nearest home until it was safe to go out again. Dumpsters on the main street were set on fire at night and people stood around them getting high and keeping warm. Hanging out 'on the strip' was the thing to do.

"Living there, we all learned that the way to earn respect from others was to make them afraid of you. That was how you 'got your juice.' Violence, burglary, and murder were every day occurrences and most of the crimes never even made the newspapers. Two of my friends were shot and killed driving down the street. The police came out only in groups of eight or ten officers when they bothered to come at all. Finally a big brick wall was built around the housing project; the politicians said it was to protect the low-income citizens from drug dealers and criminals, but the residents felt it was just the whites protecting their own and trying to keep the criminals where they belonged, with the poor.

"Did you have a job after school?" Rick asked. "What did you do for money?"

"My freshman year in high school I worked at a large grocery store called Earle's Market with a group of my friends. I was assigned to the produce and dairy sections that had coolers, and we sneaked beer into them and drank it on our breaks.

"With the money my friends and I earned, we bought new clothes and shared them since we wore about the same size. I was taller and thinner than the others, but I made adjustments so that things looked like they halfway fit. If the pants were too short, I wore them down on my hips and my shirt on the outside. Or if the shirt was too big I left the top few buttons undone and wore it open with a T-shirt underneath, like I was styling it."

"That makes me think of the hand-me-down clothes your mom brought you from work; they didn't fit right either, did they?"

"You're right. But this time at least I got to choose what to wear. Sometimes my buddies made cracks at me, saying I was so skinny I could hula-hoop through a Cheerio. Or they'd ask me if I was kin to Popeye's girlfriend, Olive Oyl. Although it hurt my feelings, I laughed with them and gradually learned that if I made fun of myself, other people wouldn't. I understood my school lessons, but my grades were average or below, which got me in trouble at home.

"Like I had done as a kid when I was sent to the closet, I still made pictures in my head of how other people lived and imagined having the love and support I saw in my friends' families. I now know I was comparing the way I was feeling on the inside, to the way other people looked on the outside, and I always came up short.

"It seemed to me that other families always stood together and defended each other from outsiders, even though they'd fight among themselves. I didn't have that kind of home, but the friends I hung with formed a kind of protective group, so in a way we were like a big family. But still, I was always jealous of everybody. I was afraid of getting into fights or doing or saying the wrong thing or being in the wrong place, afraid that I was too tall and skinny, and so ugly that nobody would want me."

"Did you play basketball? You must have."

"Yeah, I did. And I loved it—played my freshman and sophomore years and it really helped me become more confident. Finally my height turned into an asset. I was on the first string and at 6'4" I was one of the shorter team members and was the ball handler. I started feeling like I fit in, especially when I was drinking. I also learned that when I gave away enough alcohol and pot, others liked having me around.

"Basketball—it was such a high. I was part of the team. I belonged. I looked forward to practicing every day, because I was really a part of the group. Our coach was Mr. Smith, who we called Coach Sticky because he was always saying, 'Stick to your man, stick to your man.' Besides teaching us how to play the game, he taught us real teamwork, how sometimes you have to sacrifice your goals for the sake of the group. And that practice and hard work lead to success, that it's important to keep on trying no matter what. He always expected the best from us so that's what we gave him.

"At school, the team was in the limelight and we walked through the halls whenever we pleased. I was in and out of trouble for not doing my homework and for playing around when I bothered to come to class. But one of my teachers covered for me when I came in drunk. She'd even let me stay in her room till I came out of it."

"Today we call that enabling," Rick said.

"Yeah, yeah, I know," I said, shifting in my seat. "But I thought it was great at the time. It was easy for me to buy alcohol, so sometimes during the week I'd get a half a gallon of wine and a half a gallon of gin, and my friends and I would skip school and party all day at my house. We were careful to clean up before my mom came home so she wouldn't catch on, but sometimes the neighbors told her they'd seen us. If she asked me if I'd gone to school when I hadn't, I always said yes. Then she'd yell at me, 'You lying motherfucker! Don't you never bring any of your no-good friends into my fucking house when I'm not here.' She'd pick up an ashtray or glass or whatever was handy and throw it at me."

"You were drinking pretty regularly by this time?"

"Yeah. Oh, yeah. And every payday Friday all of us guys working at Earle's Market still went out and bought our new clothes, but by this time we also pooled our money and bought half a gallon of liquor so we could party that night. In addition, I always bought myself a six-pack to take home and drink while I was dressing, so by the time I met the other guys it took just a few more drinks for me to become the life or the embarrassment of the party, often the two in succession. By the end of the night I was usually falling down drunk and throwing up. Eventually the other guys got fed up with me and wouldn't let me wear their clothes because I ruined so many of them.

"When I was a junior, during the months before basketball season I went to class from seven in the morning to one in the afternoon and then worked at Columbia Yachts after school from three till midnight, five days a week. My mom never asked me to help with the bills, and I never offered. All my money went for new clothes, drinking and partying."

"Did you ever get active in the civil rights movement?" Rick asked.

I shook my head. "I'm ashamed to say no, but I didn't. Sometimes we talked about it, or argued about what should be done. I think we wanted to be a part of changing things, but we didn't know what to do, besides talk about it. Deep down I thought that Stokely Carmichael had the right approach, talking about education, but when I was with people who thought Malcolm X and his idea of using violence was the way to go, I acted like I agreed. We'd raise our fists and shout, 'Black power!' We'd light dumpsters on fire in the projects and hang around saying, 'Fuck you, Whitey!' and 'I'm black and I'm proud! Say it loud!'

"Martin Luther King's approach was less popular with the young folks because they thought nonviolent means would take too long. The old folks liked King more. To tell the truth, I never felt a part of the Civil Rights Movement, in fact, aside from the ball team I'd never felt a part of anything at all."

"Tell me about the girls in high school."

"I went out with a few girls, but not a lot. The one I liked most was Bett Jones. We ended up getting married when I got back from Vietnam, and legally, I'm still married to her but I haven't seen her in years. Back in high school she was tall and beautiful, one of the cheerleaders at our basketball games. She was always on the honor roll and could sing and dance like a professional. I thought we made a great looking pair.

"When we went out, Bett had to get dressed at a girlfriend's house because her dad was very strict. He would have blown a gasket if he'd seen her clothes. She often wore an afro wig, along with tight bell-bottom jeans that showed her navel. I'd wear my pants low on my hips, along with platform shoes, for what reason I have no idea. I already towered over everybody else, and with the added height I had to watch out for ceiling fans, sometimes even ceilings. I had the biggest Afro you'd ever want to see. The Jacksons had nothing on me. My hair stood out from shoulder to shoulder and was as tall as it was wide. I had all these outfits, bright yellow, pink, or fire engine red, you name it.

Rick and I both laughed. "I'd like to have seen that," he said. "I'll bet people remembered you!"

"They did. But that can be good or bad."

"So, back to Bett."

"Well, like I said, her father was a preacher, and they were middle class, not poor like us. I learned later that Bett's grandfather had been an alcoholic and her dad swore that he would never drink, and neither would anybody in his family. Especially Bett. She was his favorite. He didn't like me from the start and he told me if there was ever any drinking, or if I brought her in late, he wouldn't let her see me again.

"Bett never drank when we went out, but I always did. At first I made sure to follow his rules to get Bett home on time, but that didn't last. He'd restrict her for a week or two when we were late, but we'd sneak around behind his back and go out anyway.

"I'd told my mom and Ivy about this respectable, popular girl I was dating, but they didn't believe me. Finally, one Sunday I took Bett to church so my mom and her friends could see how I was moving up in the world. I have to say they were impressed for once, and they were nice to Bett.

Good Choices

✦

1998

Rick ran our last group therapy session. Like the counselors had done in other treatment centers I'd been through, he went around the room and pointed out what he saw as each individual's strengths and weaknesses. He warned every man what pitfalls to watch out for and predicted how we'd make it on the outside. I sat there and listened, as I had in other treatment programs. When he came to me, he said he had no opinion on how I would do. I remembered telling him about what the other counselors had said about me in the past, but still didn't know what to think. In a way I was hurt that he'd left me out.

Some months later I ran into him in the cafeteria, and said, "Hey, Rick, you remember the last group meeting we had?"

"Yeah," he said, tilting his head.

"Well, I just wanted to know why you didn't tell me how you thought I'd do after I got out of treatment. You remember that?"

"Sure I do," he said. "You'd told me when you came in that the counselors always thought you'd make it, and you always went back out. I didn't want to do the same thing they'd done because it was clear it hadn't helped."

"Thanks, man," I said, giving him a hug. "Thanks. I think maybe it worked."

After I completed the substance abuse program I had to wait thirty days for an opening in the PTSD Program. I made arrangements to have the tumor on my jaw removed, and I was a little apprehensive about the procedure. Mr. C., the program coordinator, helped me make a list of questions to ask the doctor. There was one I was embarrassed to ask, but he told me that no question is a stupid question. My mom always said if they operate on you, air can get into your body and kill you. When I asked the doctor, he didn't laugh or anything, just told me that wasn't true, which put my mind at ease. And the tumor turned out to be benign, nothing to worry about, just like the male nurse had thought.

While recovering from the surgery I kept busy, helping the hospital staff transport patients, reading all the recovery literature I could get my hands on, and trying to apply the lessons I'd learned in treatment. Lady G., the dom director, gave me videos by the Evangelist T.D. Jakes and some other tapes on addiction, and I spent hours watching them.

AA members in the area held meetings in the hospital twice each week, for the benefit of the patients and I attended them all. There was one man, a Vietnam vet named Patrick, who always brought one of the graduates from the substance abuse program. Patrick was a tall, handsome man who looked like a professional and usually wore a suit to the meetings. He was positive and jovial and seemed like a genuinely happy man. He was always saying, "If you haven't got a sponsor, get a sponsor." Each time he spoke, he ended with, "If nobody's told you today that they love you, I love you. Just keep coming back and fulfill the purpose God intended for you."

I really liked what Patrick said and wanted to ask him to be my sponsor, but I'd heard it was best to choose someone with a similar background because it would be easier to relate to them. Patrick was a successful white businessman from a middle class family. He'd never been to prison or lived on the streets. All we seemed to have in common were our alcoholism and Vietnam experience, but I could relate to everything he said and I respected his sobriety.

After thinking long and hard about it, I finally decided to ask him to sponsor me anyway. He had the kind of sobriety I wanted, and I thought he could help me keep from going back to where I'd been. I wanted to learn from someone who had done things right and who enjoyed life. One night after the meeting, I screwed up my courage, pulled him aside and said, "I'd like to talk to you for a minute."

"Sure," he said, and we walked over to a corner of the room.

I took a deep breath and asked, "I want to know, um, would you consider being my sponsor?"

He smiled. "I sure would," he said, and gave me a hug.

I felt like a little kid who'd just won first prize in a contest. I said, "Wait right there. I have to get something." I ran back to my room and grabbed some pages from the legal pad I'd been using to work on my twelve steps. When I got back to him, I held them out and said, "Here's my first three steps."

"Whoa," Patrick said. He laughed and held up his hands. "Wait a minute here. We've got lots of time. Let's start by going to some meetings together and getting to know each other first."

"You don't want my steps?"

"Yes, but not now. Later."

"Okay," I said, a little disappointed. I folded the papers and shoved them in my back pocket. "That's cool."

"I'll pick you up tomorrow night and take you to a meeting. I'll be here about 7:45."

"I'll be ready," I said.

Patrick took me to meetings three or four times a week, where he introduced me to lots of people. I hadn't known such a caring and loving man since I'd left the guys in Vietnam. Patrick never judged me, and he repeatedly went out of his way to be available for me. He'd call and say, "I'll pick you up at 6:30 for a meeting."

If I answered, "Oh, man, I don't know. I'm really tired."

He'd say, "Good. I'll pick you up at 6:30."

We often went out to dinner and we laughed a lot. If I didn't have any money, Patrick paid. When he saw that I didn't know how to order in nice restaurants, he ordered first so I could see how to do it. He never told me what to do, but when I had questions he gave me examples of how he'd handled similar situations. Sometimes I understood right away what he meant, and other times I didn't. But he always ended with, "Go on and try that out. Just have fun with it." I quickly grew to trust him.

After we'd been working together for a couple of months, Patrick said, "Eugene, I want you to write out a list of things you want to accomplish in the next five years."

"Like what?" I said. "You mean like how much money I want to be making? Or what kind of job I'll have?"

"Yeah, like that. And anything else you want to have by the time you're five years sober."

"Okay," I said. "I can do that."

"Then, when you've got it done, seal it up in an envelope and don't look at it till your fifth anniversary."

"Five years? All right," I said. "Hope I don't lose it."

"You'll be amazed," he said, "at where you'll be five years from now. Truly amazed."

◆   ◆   ◆

I started hanging out with one of the other patients, a guy who had studied some Eastern philosophy and called himself "Tai." He had applied for disability and was waiting to get a huge check for all the years he'd been eligible but hadn't received anything. We talked a lot about what alcohol had done to our lives. Sometimes we'd go out to eat, or drive up to his place in Dunedin, about twenty miles away.

Most of the dom patients got regular weekend passes to go home, but since I had no family or friends around, I used mine to go to lots of AA meetings. Eventually Patrick and I started a new Tuesday night meeting at the hospital, called "Vets for Sobriety."

I never missed going to the nearby Log Cabin AA meeting on Sunday nights. I'd check out one of the bikes the hospital had for patients, or I'd walk there. One day I was surprised to see one of the women from the meeting serving food in the hospital cafeteria. Cathy was tall and pretty, with long red hair. She and her mom, who was also in the program, were always at the meeting.

"Hello there," I said.

She smiled and nodded back to me.

I didn't say anything else, just moved on down the line, because I didn't want to give away her anonymity.

At 6:00 the following morning, I was outside in the gazebo, doing my morning meditation, when Cathy came over. "Hi," she said. "I'm just on my way into work."

I stood up. "Hello."

"I just wanted to let you know if there's any AA literature you'd like to have I'll be glad to get it for you."

"Thanks," I said as she turned to leave. "Appreciate it." I couldn't help but admire her figure as she walked away.

There was an AA picnic the next weekend, and I'd been invited to go with Sally and Joe, a couple in the program. It just so happened that Sally was Cathy's sponsor, and Cathy spent most of the afternoon with us. I was pretty sure she liked me, and was painfully aware of the prejudice she might encounter if we got together, a white woman with a black man. I decided then, that if we were together and people started treating her differently because of the color of my skin, I'd need to let her go. I'd never want to do anything to hurt her.

After the meeting the next Sunday night, Cathy said, "I noticed you're riding a bike. That's a pretty long ride in the dark. Can I give you a lift home?" I was really pleased that she seemed to like me, and as I threw my bike in the back of her pickup, I reminded myself that I was still in treatment and not ready for a relationship. But being with her sure felt good.

Facing the Pain

◆

1998

When it was time to enter the PTSD program and work on recovering from the ordeal I'd endured in Vietnam, I moved out of the dom and into to the third floor of Building One along with fourteen other men. We were all between forty-five and fifty-five years old, and were war veterans, mostly from Vietnam. As in the drug treatment program, we were from different branches of the service. Over half of us were on the verge of losing jobs or families, or becoming homeless.

Again, we were given full medical and psychological exams and were re-evaluated for medications. I was placed on an antidepressant and given medication for high blood pressure. But the most helpful prescription was one that let me sleep for four hours straight without the terrible nightmares I'd endured for twenty-eight years. The doctor told me the experiences I'd been calling nightmares weren't really dreams at all. I was actually re-living the awful traumas I'd been through. But we still called them nightmares.

All the PTSD staff members were veterans themselves or had a close family member who was a vet, which I thought made a lot of sense. I saw a psychiatrist every week for a medication check and a psychologist for individual therapy. A different PTSD psychologist led the group therapy. We carefully advanced through each of the three phases of the program, first working on the past, then looking at the present before moving on to the future.

At our first group meeting, we went around the room and every man gave his name, his nickname from Vietnam, his military rank and present position. Then we each talked about a past situation we'd found hard to cope with.

A lieutenant named Matt told us about the last operation he'd led in Vietnam. As a squad leader, he took ten men into the bush, and only he and one other man returned. For decades he was overcome by guilt because he hadn't been able to save those other men.

Leon said he'd come back from an R&R break in Thailand and it was his turn to "walk point" on his next mission. That is, he was to be the first one in the group to walk into the jungle, which meant if they ran into trouble he'd be the first to get hit. This common practice was intended to get Leon back into survival mode after his leave. He was still pretty shaky that day so his best friend offered to take his place. When his buddy was killed, Leon was devastated. He'd always felt it should have been him. For the remainder of his tour he volunteered to walk point on every dangerous mission he could, but he was never hit.

Gary was unable to say a word that first night, and in fact, didn't talk in the group for two weeks. The psychologist told us that his helicopter had blown up underneath him, and he was the only survivor out of twenty-three men.

The knot in my gut got tighter and tighter as we went around the room, coming closer to my turn. I told them that the name I'd gone by in Vietnam was Tree, or Treetop and talked first about being a dispatcher. My voice broke when I described the screams of terrified men who were injured or dying, and my feelings of desperation at being completely helpless to do anything to help them. And I told them about Samuels pushing me out of the helicopter and how I'd survived for three days hiding alone in the jungle.

During the first week of the program we lost two of our group members. One was caught using drugs and the other decided he wasn't ready to go through the program. That left us with thirteen, and at our next meeting we chose a name for our group, as was the custom. As a tribute to Matt, I suggested that we called ourselves "Thirteen In, Thirteen Out," meaning that we'd all hang together no matter what. And we all made it through.

Although I had individual meetings with a psychologist, the group therapy sessions helped me the most. We learned to support each other by never saying, "You shouldn't feel that way," but instead saying something like, "Everything that happened there is yours. It's real." We never tried to solve another man's problems. We talked about our feelings and learned to look at things from different perspectives. We were encouraged to accept the fact that whatever happened was over, and we had a right to feel however we felt. Our feelings were *always* validated.

We talked about the way the war protestors treated us when we came home, how they held rallies, wore T-shirts with dead babies on them, yelled insults at us, threw things, and even tried to spit on us. We all remembered being shocked at how inaccurate the news reports from Vietnam were. One of the things that bothered me most was how the comedians made jokes about Dap. I saw the Dap as something almost sacred, something that bonded soldiers together during the most terrifying experiences of our lives, and people were making fun of it.

We tried to understand where the protestors were coming from in their opposition to the war. They encouraged us to accept the fact that we had resentments but to understand that we did not have to let those feelings control our behavior.

It was very intense and emotional, particularly during "Grief Week," which was about halfway through treatment. When they told us we'd be watching film footage of battles in Vietnam, I immediately thought of the one I'd seen at the V.A. in Hampton; the one I had to leave because I was sure I'd heard my own voice as the dispatcher. At first I didn't think I could go through that again. If that's what it took it was all over. I'd rather die. But as the days passed, I got to know the others and I realized we all felt the same way. They really understood. I wouldn't be alone this time like I'd been in Hampton.

Watching the film was horrible; I hope I never have to see anything like that again. I was drenched in sweat, my stomach in knots, consumed with fear. Unable to stop the tears, I grabbed a handful of tissues from a nearby box. Seeing wounded men screaming, helicopters crashing and exploding into flames, men running, crying, dying brought back all the things we'd faced while we were there.

While the film was running I became aware of the faces of the other men in the room. Some were crying, sobbing without trying to hide it, others had panicky looks on their faces but were still trying to hold it in. A few looked stonefaced, numb. Watching it together, confronting the past with these men, the past I'd run from for almost thirty years was, for me, a huge step toward healing.

We saw other movies of vets talking about their time in Vietnam, and how hard it was to adjust when they returned home because they hadn't gone through any "de-briefing" process as soldiers from other wars had routinely done.

Grief Week seemed to be the turning point. Most of us had closed off the war in our own minds, stuffed it down inside ourselves and never "went there." Being with a group of men who'd had similar experiences was comforting for all of us. We were with people who understood in a way others couldn't.

We learned that when soldiers from other wars get together, at Veterans of Foreign Wars (VFW) Halls or at reunions, they talk about their war experiences. But when Vietnam vets get together, they give each other the Dap handshake, and in that way recognize their common experience, but they almost never talk about the war.

During a therapy session with the psychologist, I told her about the worst recurring nightmare I kept having. She said, "All right, Tree, let's work on that. I want you to try something."

"Okay," I said.

"Remember a wound you had a long time ago. Something that really hurt, like a bad accident or a fall."

One immediately came to mind. "Okay," I said. "I've got one. It happened when I was ten. I was running with some other kids through a field of high weeds and I tripped and cut my hand on a beer bottle. I couldn't believe all the blood I saw and I was scared to death. My friends freaked out and that scared me even more. When I got home, my mom couldn't stop the bleeding, so she ended up taking me to the hospital where they admitted me for a couple of days. I went to physical therapy for a while after that, but I never did get back the full use of my little finger." I held it up and tried to bend it, for the psychologist to see.

"Okay," she said. "Now look at the scar. Remember how it hurt. Really think about it, because that hurt is yours. You own it. It's all right to feel whatever you feel."

I looked at my hand. I remembered how scared I was, and how afraid I was to go home because I knew my mom would be mad. Gradually, I felt the fear and the pain again.

"You've been trying to deny your feelings, blaming yourself for being what you think of as weak. But it isn't weak to feel your feelings. You can release yourself from the pain of the past. You can let it go."

I looked up at her, then back down to my hand.

"Now, remember how it healed," she said. "Remember how you had to be careful of it, to keep it clean and dry, not to bump it or make it worse."

I thought of the bulky white bandage wrapped around my entire hand and how I always seemed to be hitting it on something. At first the pain was so sharp it had made me cry. Then I recalled the weeks of physical therapy. It hurt a lot in the beginning, but slowly my hand got better.

"Now," she said, "look at that place today. You can still see it, and you can remember the hurt and the pain. That's yours, that hurt and pain."

I looked at her. "I see it. I remember."

"But today it isn't hurting. *Today* it isn't hurting. *Today it isn't hurting!*"

I looked back at my hand. Something clicked in my head. That exercise gave me a different perspective on what I'd been through and showed me a new way to deal with my past. I learned that it was all right for me to remember the war. I didn't have to run from it anymore. But I didn't have to keep living it every day, either. It made sense. I was no longer there. The fear and pain faded.

◆   ◆   ◆

Another step in changing my life meant taking responsibility for my past behavior, which, at that point, meant sending my father another letter. This time I wrote about the things I hadn't done rather than the things I'd done wrong. I told him I wanted to make amends to him, to set things right. I said that I wished I'd followed more of his advice and gotten more involved with the family; I wished I'd been able to get to know him better.

I also wrote to Bett, who I was still legally married to, and to my daughters, Puff and Kelsey.

There was another person I wanted to make amends to, but I didn't know her name. One Sunday, probably ten years before, when I was really sick from using heroin, I borrowed a car, parked it behind a grocery store, and waited. When an older woman came around the corner, holding her purse by the handle, I ran over and grabbed it and at the same time pushed her away. I still remember the sickening thud as she hit the ground, and I'd always felt bad that I'd done that. To make amends to her I took thirty dollars, the amount I'd stolen from her, put it in an envelope addressed to God, and dropped it in a mailbox. I thought about donating the money to some good cause, or buying someone something with it, but in the end I decided to let God decide where that money ended up.

◆   ◆   ◆

By this time everybody was calling me Tree and the name stuck, just like it had in Vietnam. I'd learned to express my fears and thoughts more openly, with the honest desire to seek the help I needed and be ready to accept it. I continued to put suggestions into action and my life changed.

The last program I wanted to complete at the V.A. was The Compensated Work Therapy Program (CWT). It would give me a chance to work and earn enough money to get on my feet while I was still a patient, living at the hospital. During the two-month wait to get in, I once again volunteered to help with other patients and attended every AA meeting I could.

Cathy kept offering me rides back to the dom, and I always took her up on it. One week she rode a bike to the meeting. "Would you mind riding part of the way home with me?" she asked. "There's a few blocks that go through a really dark area, and I'd feel safer if you were with me."

"Sure," I said, feeling very pleased. "I can do that."

We spoke a little as we rode along, and after going a mile or so, came to a small park with several benches. "Let's stop here for a few minutes," Cathy said. "We can visit for a while."

We walked our bikes down a winding sidewalk and sat on a bench by a small lake. She turned to me. "I really like the things you say in the meetings. Sounds like you've been through a lot in your life."

"I guess so," I said. "But I don't know a lot about you. Tell me about yourself."

"Well, I'm divorced," she said, "and I have one son and a grandson."

"A grandchild? You don't look old enough."

"I'm a very young grandmother," she said, and laughed. "Of course." She flipped her long red hair over her shoulder. "And you've met my mom. We live together over on the beach."

"Nice," I said. "How long have you been in the program?"

"About six months. Not much different from you."

We talked on about the program, how it had helped us, and about ourselves. She moved a little closer and I put my arm around her. As we stood up to leave, I leaned down and kissed her lightly.

I didn't have a year in the program yet, and Patrick had warned me about getting into a relationship too soon. Before that kiss was even over, I'd reminded myself that my sobriety came first, and I needed to talk to Patrick. I told Cathy she should talk to her sponsor too, because she didn't have a year in the program either. But as I rode the rest of the way back to the dom, I was pleased and at the same time a little nervous.

She rode her bike again the next week and after the meeting we both headed straight for the park without either of us mentioning it. When we got to "our" bench, the conversation didn't last long. I'd been thinking about her all week and could hardly control myself. Seemed to me she felt the same. I pulled her close and we kissed eagerly. Then I pulled back.

"Maybe we'd better …" I was gasping for breath. "I mean …"

"No, no, we don't have to stop," she said, drawing me back to her.

I kissed her again and then moved away. "I don't want to, Cathy, but I think we'd better stop." I could tell by her face that I'd offended her. "Please don't be hurt or mad. I just want to do the right thing."

"Is it me? Is something wrong with me?"

"No, no, Cathy. I don't want to stop. But I'm not going to get involved any further till I talk to my sponsor."

"What does he have to do with this?"

"I have too much to lose, Cathy. I've worked too hard to get this far and I'm not taking any chances on losing it."

She looked at me as she straightened her blouse. "We're not hurting anything."

"Please believe me, Cathy. I just need to talk to Patrick."

◆   ◆   ◆

I was at a meeting with Patrick the following week when I told him that I wanted to start seeing Cathy.

He said, "You need to get to know yourself first, Eugene. Other relationships are a helluva lot easier when you have a good relationship with yourself."

"Okay," I said.

"You've been working a great program. I've noticed that some of the women have been checking you out—like Cathy."

I just smiled.

"Now, I'm talking as your sponsor. You seem to think you're ready for a relationship, so I know you must be horny. And I have someone in mind for you."

I looked at him, puzzled, and thought, *Do sponsors do that?*

"I believe I know you pretty well," Patrick said, "and I figure you want someone you wouldn't mind waking up with in the morning. Is that right?"

"Yeah," I said.

"I figure you'd want someone you could take to dinner and to the movies, maybe go for long walks on the beach."

"Yeah, yeah," I said, smiling. "You know me pretty good, all right."

"Well, I'd like to introduce you if I may," he said.

"Yes, yes, yes," I said, looking around for someone.

"Eugene," Patrick said, "I'd like to introduce you to Eugene."

"What?" I didn't understand.

He laughed. "The first year is a time for you to build a relationship with yourself and a higher power. I want you to do those things with yourself."

So, I took myself to dinners and went on long walks on the beach, and gradually I began to like the person I woke up with every morning. Me.

Telling on Myself

✦

1998

Although I was feeling good about the way things were going, there was a secret that I hadn't told anyone, not even Patrick, because I was afraid he might not want to continue to sponsor me. But I knew I had to tell him. I'd heard too many times that keeping secrets could lead me back to drinking and drugging, and for me that would be a death sentence. I knew I had to get this done before I started the CWT Work Program.

Patrick and I were driving home from a meeting one night when I took a deep breath and thought to myself, *This is the time. I have to do it now.* It took every bit of courage I had to say, "Patrick, there's something I haven't told you."

"What's that?" he said, glancing over at me.

"I've got an outstanding warrant in Tampa."

"Yeah?" he said, without even hesitating. "What for?"

"It's an old trespassing charge. I just quit reporting to my probation officer." I looked over at him, but he was focused on the road ahead. "I saw her the day I got out of jail after my mom died, and I paid her my fifteen dollars. But then I left town and I just never contacted her again."

"Okay," Patrick said.

I hated having to tell him, but once I got started, it felt good to finally talk about it. "I already know the only way I can clear it up is to turn myself in. I'll have to stay in jail till the hearing, but that doesn't bother me. What scares me is that the V.A. might not let me in the CWT."

"Well …" Patrick said.

"When I filled out their application, I wrote down the old warrants I knew were still out in Virginia, but nothing in Tampa."

"Well, now," he said, looking over at me. "You gotta do something about that."

"Yeah, I know. I know I do," I said, looking down at my knees.

"You have to do the right thing. And however things work out will be God's will."

"I know," I said. "You're right."

"I'll stand right beside you while you go through it," he said, reaching over and grabbing my shoulder.

The relief I felt was tremendous. I was almost light-hearted. Somebody had my back. I wasn't alone.

After talking to Patrick, I had a little more confidence. I reminded myself that I'd been a model patient. I had no infractions against me, I'd been helpful, willing, and was always doing something positive. The next day I told Mr. C. what I'd done, and he understood. So did my counselors, every single one. Even the medical director for the domiciliary said, "Eugene, you just do whatever you need to do, and I promise when you finish, whatever sentence you get, we'll find room for you here." I could hardly believe my ears. It was working. I'd been honest and made the responsible decision, although it was hard to do. Instead of running away, I faced the things that really scared me and people didn't desert me.

I called the probation officer I'd last seen eight months before. She said, "You need to come to my office this afternoon at 3:30. I'll have the police here to arrest you."

My heart sank, but I knew I was doing the right thing. "All right," I said. "I'll be there."

That afternoon Patrick drove me over to her office and the police took me to jail. They checked me in and put me in an orange jump suit that was two sizes too wide and two sizes too short. To my surprise, for the first time in thirty years I was frightened and unsure of myself in jail. Every other time, within an hour or so I fit right in with all the other inmates, but this time I just couldn't get comfortable. In the past I was glad to get the food, but now I could hardly make myself eat.

When I went in the courtroom the following morning, I was surprised to see Patrick and Tai there. Patrick waved. When they called my name, I went up and the judge glanced down at me and said, "So, you turned yourself in? Was it cold out there?"

I looked at him but didn't answer, and he set a court date for two weeks later. As I was leaving, I looked back and Patrick waved again.

When we returned to the jail the nurse told me they wouldn't give me any of my medication but the blood pressure pills, which was bad news. It meant I wouldn't be sleeping again till I got out.

During the two weeks I waited for the hearing, I tried to go to those faraway places in my mind, the ones I'd visited when I was a kid locked in the closet, and later when I was on the streets, but I couldn't do it any more. After being able to sleep through the night, having to face those horrible nightmares again, waking up screaming and covered in sweat, was unbearable.

I was really worried about the sentence I might get and did my best to trust that things would turn out the way they were supposed to, like Patrick said. But fear kept creeping in. If I had to stay in jail for a year there was no way they could hold the dom room for me. When I got out I'd be back on the streets. I'd be a dead man.

While I was there I wrote to Patrick, but at his suggestion I didn't bring Cathy's address with me. I wasn't expecting any letters and was really surprised when I heard my name at mail call. I was even more surprised to get a note from Cathy. I wrote back to her about getting clean and sober and about seeing her when I got out, but I told her I wasn't going to let anyone or anything come between me and my sobriety. I told her I'd be checking with my sponsor and reminded her to check with hers. But I was really grateful to get some mail.

I met my lawyer for the first time just before my hearing, but I knew how the system worked before I even talked to him. The judge could order me to serve the rest of my one-year sentence or he could put me back on probation. The lawyer didn't even ask me anything, just said, "When we go in, sit on one of the benches to the judge's left. Then when they call your name, come up and stand beside me. The judge will read the charges and I'll answer him. He'll sentence you and that'll be the end of it."

"Can't I say something?"

"No, you don't need to. You look to be in pretty good shape," he said, and walked over to one of the other prisoners.

I can't say anything? I thought. *I'm fucked. I should be able to speak in my own defense. Fucking lawyer. It's all over.*

The hallway was full of activity, people talking and moving around. Finally the bailiff called us all in and we walked to the area the lawyer had mentioned. I just kept my head down till they called my name. Then I went over to stand by the lawyer, just like he'd told me to.

"Your Honor," the lawyer said, "This man voluntarily turned himself in for a probation violation. He wants to clear up whatever obligations he has to the City of Tampa and the court system. He's throwing himself on the mercy of the court. And I have to say he has a lot of supporters." The lawyer turned around and pointed to the back of the room. "I must say, Judge, with this much backing, I think he has a good chance of making it."

The judge looked to the back of the room and said, "Stand up, all of you who are here for Mr. Hairston."

I turned around and saw Patrick and Tai smiling and waving at me. And there must have been twelve other people standing with them, including Mr. C., Lady G., the social worker, counselors from the SATP and PTSD programs, the Assistant Director of the PTSD program, an AA member who was an attorney, and the rest were from the Log Cabin AA group. Tears came to my eyes. I was overcome with gratitude. I'd never imagined there were so many people who cared so much about me.

"My, Mr. Hairston, you have quite an entourage here," the judge said. "I understand some of them are your therapists from your treatment program. And I've been getting letters about you from all kinds of people."

I smiled at him in surprise, daring to hope that things might work out.

"With this many people ready to help you, I see no reason to return you to jail. While technically, I'm placing you on continued probation with the condition that you complete your V.A. programs, there will be no need to report back to your probation officer. You'll be released today, and you can start anew."

Tears rolled down my cheeks. "Thank you, Judge," I said. "Thank you, sir." A heavy weight lifted from my shoulders as I returned to my seat, smiling broadly at all my friends in the back of the room.

We left the courtroom about 11:30 and on my way out, Tai came over and said, "I'll wait for you, man. I'll take you back to Bay Pines."

"Cool," I said.

By the time they processed me out of the ward, and then out of the jail, it was 6:30 p.m. I didn't expect Tai to have waited all that time, but he was sitting right next to the exit. He came up and gave me a big hug, and as we walked out I recognized that once again, I'd faced my fears and everything worked out. I had really made progress in cleaning up the wreckage of my past.

"Hungry?" Tai asked me.

"I'm starved. The food in that place sucks. Let's get some fried chicken."

◆   ◆   ◆

When I got back to the hospital, the first thing I did was go around and thank everybody who'd come to support me. I started working in the CWT Program the next day as a housekeeper in the same domiciliary I lived in, earning four hundred dollars every two weeks. Three hundred of that was deposited in a savings account so that when I left the program I'd have enough money to get housing, clothing, and other things I'd need.

When the regular housekeeping staff found out I was in the CWT Program and not a regular employee, at first some of them treated me with suspicion. A few thought I was just trying to work the system as a way to get disability. Several times, when I was working in the area with a woman I found attractive, I'd start up a conversation. One day I asked one of the file clerks if she'd like to go to a movie.

She said, "Who are you? Are you a patient?"

"No, I work here," I said.

"You CWT?" she asked?

"Well, yeah. I am," I said.

"No thanks. I don't think so."

Another woman I asked out just laughed and told me she had eleven children. Eventually I learned she wasn't lying. A year or so later, after I'd proven myself, I was told some of the women came to regret having turned me down.

But at the time, I stopped asking for dates and instead put my attention on the patients, veterans who were mostly old, sick, and grumpy. I always wore my veteran's insignia, so they'd know I was a vet like them, and did my best to cheer them up. I didn't pamper or coddle them like some of the other staff members did. Instead I'd walk in the room and say something like, "Hey, man, there's a recruiter out in the hall waiting to see you. He's looking for somebody to teach those young kids how to do things right for a change. You up for it?" When I got a chuckle or a smile out of them, I felt really good.

I volunteered for everything, coming in on Saturdays to help set up rooms for meetings, working late, taking on little jobs that nobody else wanted. When I saw something that needed to be done, I just did it, which won me accolades from the patients and my co-workers. Three months after completing the CWT program and getting hired as a housekeeper, I was promoted to work leader, where I assisted the supervisor and was responsible for distributing tasks to the other housekeepers.

Because I'd been there only a short time, some of the others resented me. I knew they didn't want me giving them instructions so I worked alongside them, volunteering to do some of the jobs they didn't want to do. When they saw me working, they began to trust me. I continued to volunteer for everything. One of the computer training educators told me that the first time she remembered seeing me I had one beeper, then a week later I had two, and a short while later, I had three. Gradually I earned a reputation for dependability and I heard the nurse managers and other staff talking among themselves, saying, "If you want something done, call Tree. He'll get to it faster than a supervisor will."

◆   ◆   ◆

On the anniversary of my first year in sobriety, I couldn't believe I'd done it. I hadn't craved a drink or drug in all that time, when for decades I couldn't even go a day without getting high. Even though for most of that year I'd been living on the grounds of the hospital, in a safe, protected environment, I'd been sober for a year.

I'll never be able to express the gratitude I felt when I took my one-year medallion from Patrick's hand at the end of the meeting on August 12, 1999. The tears wouldn't stop. When I sat back down, I couldn't stop caressing the metal coin, the size of a silver dollar, engraved with the Serenity Prayer on one side and the AA symbol on the other.

Afterward, Patrick gave me a cupcake with a big "One Year" candle stuck in it, and he took a Polaroid picture of me. When he gave me the photo, my first thought was that something didn't look right. It took me a while to figure it out, but what looked so strange was that I was smiling. I didn't smile for my mug shots. I'd never seen a picture of myself looking happy as an adult. This was not just a smile; it was a big clownish grin. I thought to myself, This must be what happiness looks like.

Since I'd completed a year in the program, I started going out with Cathy on actual dates. She'd pick me up and we'd usually go to dinner, then she'd bring me back to the dom where we'd talk. A few weeks later I got a weekend pass and rented a hotel room over on Madeira Beach.

I have to say, I was a little nervous. It had been a while since I'd been with a woman. But Cathy was wonderful. She slowly undressed me, then I removed her clothes and led her to the bed. When we made love for the first time, slow and easy, it was tender and loving, so different for me. After all those years on the streets and in institutions, I could hardly remember what it was like to be alone with someone I really cared about.

With Cathy, I found comfort. And I trusted her. I knew she wasn't trying to use me, to get something out of me; she even offered to pay for half the room and meals, although I didn't let her. With her, I didn't have to act like I was someone I wasn't. I didn't have to perform, or make sure I got what I thought I deserved, as I had in the past. We took long walks on the beach and went to eat at nice restaurants. In one way, the thought of getting into an ongoing relationship sounded great, but at the same time, commitment was something I'd learned to avoid at any cost.

◆　　　◆　　　◆

At work, Mr. C. encouraged me to apply for a full-time position, a "real" job as a Housekeeping Aide. I wanted to move up, of course, but was nervous about the fact that everybody knew my history of addiction and homelessness, and also that I'd have to include my criminal record on the application form. Mr. C. said, "Don't be afraid to put down the things from your past, Eugene. It's leaving them out that could get you into trouble."

I took his advice and sent off for my records from Virginia and Tampa. When I got my rap sheet back and showed it to my counselors, they stared at me, open-mouthed. "Is this really you?" they asked. I told myself that my record was a list of things I had done, but it was not who I was.

I got the Housekeeping Aide job and was assigned to the nursing home at the hospital, working for a different section manager and supervisor. That made me a little nervous. I'd gotten comfortable in the first job because I knew everybody, but this was something new.

I remembered that when I expressed my fears I got feedback, so I talked to Mr. C.

"You know, Eugene," he said, "maybe they want to see if you'll do as good a job there as you did in the dom." Somehow that simple statement changed the way I saw things. Taking on the new job became a goal that I wanted to achieve rather than a fear I wanted to run away from.

I'd run from challenges my whole life, but this was one I was ready for. People in recovery told me that fear was a part of life, but so long as I examined my motives and focused on doing the next right thing for the next right, good reason, that it would be enough. I reminded myself that I'd gotten a lot of compliments about my attitude and my work ethic. So I started at the nursing home, and at the age of forty-eight, I began my first legitimate career.

Again, some of the others seemed to resent my getting the job, and I heard them saying, "They just gave him that job because he was a homeless vet. He don't really deserve it," and "Why'd they promote him? I been here longer. It ain't fair." I did my best to ignore them and focus on the present as I had been taught, doing my job to the best of my ability. When I cleaned a room, I made sure I scrubbed every corner and mopped under every bed. I was cheerful with patients and co-workers, always smiling and saying hello, even to those who never answered. I did my best to be diplomatic when difficulties came up and to concentrate on being a part of the solution, not part of the problem.

After a few weeks, the thought came to me that I was working in a facility like my mom had been in when she died. By doing my best and being kind to the patients, I felt, in some small way, that I was making up for the fact that I hadn't been there for her. I consciously worked hard to make every job I did be a reflection of who I really was. It wasn't long before I received awards of appreciation from the nurses and patients, as well as my supervisors and fellow workers.

◆   ◆   ◆

I was still living at the hospital, but often spent weekends with Tai, who lived in a mobile home park in nearby Dunedin. On one of those visits I went with him to pay his rent. When we walked into the park office, the manager was sitting at her desk looking up at an elderly woman. The old lady said, "Honey, my husband died, and I'm not going to be able to come back down next year. I need to sell the place."

That sounded interesting. I was ready to get a place of my own. "Do you need a buyer?" I asked, stepping over to the desk.

She turned around and looked at me.

"I might be interested," I said. "How much you asking?"

She smiled. "Well now, it needs some repairs," she said, shaking her head a little. "Why don't you take a look at it and see what you think?" She put her purse down on the manager's desk and pulled out a key. "I just want to get rid of it, to tell you the truth. All I'm asking is five hundred dollars. Of course, you still have to rent the land. That's separate."

A home for five hundred dollars? I took the key and Tai and I went right then and looked at the place. Saying it needed a lot of work was an understatement. The flooring in both bedrooms was completely gone and spots in the living room had rotted through because the roof had a bad leak.

"Man, could we ever fix this up?" I asked Tai. "I don't know. It's a long way from the V.A. and I don't have a car."

"You'll have one before long, the way you're going," he said. "You ain't never gonna find a better deal. And you'll be living up here right near me! I'll work on it with you. We can do it!"

I decided this was just too good to pass up, so I wrote the woman a check right then and there. For the first time I had a home in my own name. For five hundred dollars. After the old lady left, I said to the manager, "I'll have to fix the place up before I can move in. So when you turn off the electricity, I'll have to get it turned back on so we can use power tools."

"No problem," she said, winking at Tai, who had been on a couple of dates with her. "I'll leave it on for a couple of months. And I'll keep the water on, too. You won't need to pay rent on the lot till you move in."

"Thank you so much." I couldn't believe my luck. "That's cool," I said.

Tai helped me work on the place every weekend. I used the money I'd saved through the CWT Program to buy the place, and for the supplies we needed to repair it. It took lots of weekends of hard work to get things into shape. Then all I needed was furniture.

As Tai and I were finishing up the painting, the manager came by to check the place out. "Listen," she said, holding out two sets of keys. "There are two homes in the park that are full of furniture and the owners aren't coming back. They told me to get rid of it, so you can go in and take whatever you want."

I was able to furnish my first home without spending a dollar. When I finally moved in, people started giving me curtains and rugs and knickknacks and such. Mr. C. gave me an entertainment center with a wide screen TV, complete with all the other contraptions, speakers, a VCR and a DVD player.

Being more than twenty miles from my job with only a bicycle for transportation was my biggest problem, but I had a plan. I got up at 4:30 each morning and rode my bike five miles to Clearwater to catch the 5:30 bus. I was able to put my bike on the front of the bus, so when I got off in St. Pete I could ride it from there to the hospital. That got me to work at seven. Then every night I did it all over again, in reverse. In the seven months I did that, before I was able to get a car, I only got rained on once.

Every night, when I walked in the door from work, I appreciated everything I had. My life was good. Sitting in the living room one afternoon, looking at my furnishings and curtains, I noticed that everything matched. It was as if I'd been working with an interior decorator. I knew in my heart that this was not just an act of people's good will. It was not only my being in the right place at the right time. There was another force at work, something much greater than all of us.

Some might think that everything happened by coincidence, but that doesn't work for me. If things hadn't happened just the way they did, I don't believe I'd be alive today. For example, that morning I woke up in the refrigerator box in Tampa, if my regular V.A. counselor had been working instead of the intern, I might not have gotten into treatment the same day. Also, I just happened to be with Tai at the mobile home park when that elderly woman came in to sell her place; and that happened when I had the money to buy it; and Tai was in town just long enough to help me fix it up. And, I met Patrick, my AA sponsor, who was always supportive, never critical, always willing to listen and never looked down on me.

I'd always believed in God, but now it seemed so very clear that there was a higher authority working in my life, something powerful and mysterious. I could see no logical, rational way to explain how, after repeatedly trying and failing to recover from decades of substance abuse, I was able to become a sober, responsible man. I wondered how many other "coincidences" or opportunities I'd been given to change my life that I just hadn't seen.

Getting sober was hard and sometimes painful, but little by little, week by week, I continued to see changes within myself. I could never have done it without the help of my higher power. I always remember the phrase, "If you take one step, God will take two." To this very day I'm conscious of that and always try to be willing to take that step.

◆   ◆   ◆

When I was able to afford a car, Cathy went with me to buy it and I ended up with an old white Oldsmobile that had no air conditioning, but it ran just fine. Cathy started coming up to Dunedin on weekends, and I stayed over with her in St. Petersburg on Wednesday nights. We went out to eat, to AA meetings and to movies. As our relationship grew, I began to feel more and more uncomfortable about making a commitment to her. In the past, my relationships with women all ended unhappily and I didn't want to get hurt again. Each time I began to pull away from her we were able to talk about it, and when I spoke to my sponsor, he said to try not to judge the present by what had happened in the past.

She was always buying me little gifts, which made me nervous. In my life, people only gave you something when they had an ulterior motive. When I'd accepted gifts, sooner or later they were used against me. One day I said, "Cathy, I want you to stop buying things for me. It's kind of you to do it, but to tell the truth, it makes me feel beholden to you, like I need to get you something."

She looked at me and tilted her head. "But I enjoy doing it. I don't want anything back from you."

"Still," I said. "I'd appreciate it if you'd stop."

"We'll see," she said. "I'm not making any promises."

She still buys me things, but I try to remember that she buys things for lots of people, not just me. She's helped me with things I'd never done, like opening a checking account, getting car insurance, and going to parties without getting drunk or high. Like Patrick, she never looked down on me just because I didn't know something. She seemed to sense when I needed her and let me know that she cared.

We talked openly about our future together, our boundaries, and what we each expected from our relationship. I told her that I was still legally married, although I hadn't seen my wife in over ten years, and divorce was probably somewhere in my future. We decided, at that point, to make our commitment to each other for one day at a time. So long as things were going well and we were both happy, we'd keep it that way. But, I told her if she found someone else, I'd understand.

Recovery has to be the most important thing in my life. It's everything to me, because without it, I have nothing. Without it, I'm a dead man walking. Sobriety will always have to come first.

Finding Eugene

✦

1999–2005

Three or four months after I took the housekeeping aide job, Mr. C. told me about another opening. "I've heard your boss is happy with your work," he said. "I think you'd have a good chance to move up. He leaned back in his chair and grinned. "You might want consider cutting your hair and going corporate."

I'd always worn my long hair pulled back and was proud of the way it looked. I didn't want to cut it, but I thought to myself, maybe someday. Just not right now.

Although I was nervous, I applied for the Housekeeper Aide 3 Work Leader position and within several weeks, was promoted. I continued with the mind-set that had worked for me of doing the best job I could every day and not worrying about what the future would bring. In less than six months I applied for a Maintenance Worker position, and advanced again, this time reporting directly to the Zone 2 Manager.

Several times staff members refused to complete an assignment I'd given them, or told me it should be done differently from what I'd directed. When that happened, I did the job myself, working right along side them, making repairs, cleaning up, or filling in wherever I was needed. I brought donuts and candy into the office for everybody. I cracked jokes and rewarded the staff for jobs well done. I learned by reading and by watching the way others supervised staff, that when I had to address an issue with someone on my team it was a good idea to mention two things the individual was doing well before bringing up the problem.

◆　　◆　　◆

As my fifth anniversary of sobriety approached, I remembered the list I'd made when I was a couple of months clean—where I'd hoped to be five years later. And the time was coming to open it. I knew right where the envelope was but couldn't remember what I'd written down. As it happened, my AA home group had a meeting on my anniversary date and I decided I'd open the envelope there and read it in front of my friends, people I'd grown to trust and to love.

As I stood in front of the group that night and tore open the envelope, my hands were shaking. Tears came to my eyes as I read the words I had written:

In five years I will:

- Have a job close to the V.A. Hospital

- Have an apartment close to work

- Live near a bus stop or have a bike to ride to work

- Have money to pay my bills each month

- Be in a relationship

I remembered being told that my life would be beyond my wildest dreams, and looking at the list, I realized it was. I had become a man with dignity and self-respect. I was comfortable in my own skin for the first time in my entire life.

In addition to that, I:

- Was an employee of Bay Pines V.A. Hospital

- Was establishing a solid credit rating since I paid my bills on time

- Owned my own home

- Owned my own car

- Was in a relationship with the love of my life

◆   ◆   ◆

Within a few days of my anniversary, Bett called me out of the blue, saying she and Kelsey were coming down to Disney World with the grandkids and she asked if I'd like to meet them one day for lunch. Immediately, I was thrown back into the old days, when I felt less than a man, full of anger and frustration and completely unable to change. Just the sound of her voice brought back the old fear and feelings of chaos. But somehow, at the same time, that old life seemed to belong to someone else.

The thought of being reunited with my daughter and visiting with grandchildren I'd never seen, was exciting. "That would be cool," I said to her. "I'd really like that."

"Okay," she said. "We're getting to Orlando next Monday and leaving Friday morning. We'll be at the Holiday Inn, so why don't you meet us for lunch on Wednesday?"

"Wednesday. I'll have to see if I can get off work. But that's probably okay."

"I'll call you when we get to Orlando and let you know where to meet us," she said in a voice that was a little too sexy. "I'm really looking forward to getting together with you."

I put the phone down, excited about seeing Kelsey and grandkids I'd never met, but not at all sure about seeing Bett. But at the same time I wanted my family to see for themselves that I'd truly changed, and that I was a good, decent man.

Bett phoned early Wednesday and said they would meet me at noon at the Chili's on International Drive in Orlando. I set out from the office in St. Pete at about 10:00, but before I even reached Interstate 4 in Tampa, the traffic was stopped dead. A semi had jack-knifed and cars were backed up for miles. There was no way I'd be able to get there by noon. I headed back to work and called Bett. She said she'd see when they could reschedule the meeting and call me back.

On Thursday morning she reached me at the office. "Hi Baby," she said. "Want to come over tomorrow? I really want to see you."

"I thought you were leaving early tomorrow," I said.

"The kids are," she said. "But I'm staying over an extra day so we can spend some time together. Just the two of us."

My stomach knotted up. "Bett," I said, "I really wanted to see the kids, and I'm disappointed I couldn't get there." I paused. "And I know this probably won't make sense to you, but I can't come over to see you. I'm … I'm a different man now. I lead a different life."

"Aw, come on, Baby. Don't you have just a little time for me? Just a little? We can catch up. Daddy even said to tell you hello. Can you believe it?"

"Bett," I started.

"I come all the way down here, you know. I really want to see you, Baby."

"Bett, I'm sorry. I really don't expect you to understand …"

"Oh, I understand all right," she said, her voice changing to the old familiar accusing tone. "I stood by you all those years. I put up with all your shit when you was nothing but a junkie, and now you think you're better than me!"

"No, Bett, that's not what I said. I just meant …"

"I heard you. I know what you said. You can just go fuck yourself." She slammed the receiver down in my ear.

I stared out the window of my office into the bright, sunny day. I was disappointed not to see Kelsey, but at the same time I was relieved. Seeing her would bring back all the shame of my old life, all the years when my girls had seen me belittled and humiliated by others. I had not been a good husband or father and I could not change the past. But I told myself I'd visit them some day in the future.

Not long after, I filed for divorce and it was final within the year.

◆   ◆   ◆

The following week, my Zone Manager had to take extended sick leave and I was asked to do her job temporarily. I filled in for three months without a pay increase, since she was planning to come back. When she decided to retire, I was promoted to that position. Not long after, I got that haircut.

There have been challenges to face in each new job. When I became Zone 2 Manager, once again some people were angry because they had more seniority and felt they were more qualified. As I'd done before, I concentrated on doing the next right thing every day and tried to ignore what other people might have been thinking. I always attended AA meetings regularly, and at one of them I heard somebody say, "It's none of my business what other people think about me." That made good sense. That helped.

I focused on encouraging the staff and talked to them about wiping the slate clean when they came to our team. They could leave the problems they had in other positions behind them and start anew. I spoke with them individually about their career goals and helped several of them make major improvements in their attitudes that led to promotions. One of them, a disgruntled man who had worked at the hospital for twenty years, was considered incorrigible. I treated him just as I had everyone else, and we worked together to improve his attitude and self-esteem. After a time he changed so much that he was able to advance to the position he'd always wanted.

◆   ◆   ◆

In the old days, my rap sheet was a summary of my actions. If I'd gone back to prison one more time, I'd have been designated a career criminal and would have received a mandatory life sentence.

My old record included:

- 3 armed robberies
- 2 midnight burglaries
- numerous assaults
- assault with a deadly weapon
- numerous shoplifting offenses
- felony petty theft
- numerous charges for possession of drugs
- numerous charges for possession of drugs with intent to sell
- possession of drugs with intent to sell with a firearm
- resisting arrest
- eluding police arrest and capture
- numerous parole and probation violations
- trespassing

Today, I have a very different kind of record. My resume reads:

- Zone 2 Manager
- Assistant Training Officer for Facility Support
- Member of the Hazardous Materials Weapons of Mass Destruction First Response Team/Bay Pines V.A. Medical Center and the State of Florida
- Graduate of the Veteran's Integrated Service Network (VISN) Competency Development Leadership Program
- The first CWT Graduate of the hospital's STEP Leadership Training
- Author of a training module featured on the V.A.'s Virtual Learning Center that led to a reduction of cross-contamination of the potentially dangerous C-Diff bacteria, common in hospitals and nursing homes. That training has been recommended to V.A. Hospitals across the United States.
- Author of an innovative computer training program that enables staff to earn credits for computer courses

- Member of the following committees:
  - Infection Control (Appointed by the Associate Director)
  - Patient Care Discharge
  - Incentive Awards
  - Safety
  - National Emergency Response Roster
  - Equipment
- Co-leader of Bay Pines Heart Walk Foundation
- Recipient of the Department of Veteran's Affairs Secretary's Hero Award, one of the highest awards given, for work done with Hurricane Katrina victims
- Creator of "Tree's Corner," a weekly inspirational newsletter for hospital staff

When I look at this list of accomplishments, I can hardly believe it myself.

The Calm After the Storm

◆

2005

In September 2005, I was in Phoenix, Arizona, at the 20th Anniversary Conference and Technical Exhibition of the American Society for Healthcare Environmental Services (ASHES). It was my very first national conference. I was proud to have been asked to speak to V.A. executives, but at the same time, I was scared half to death. I was slated to present an effective training project I'd created for the hospital housekeeping staff, and I'd practiced my speech at least a hundred times. This opportunity was a real high point for me, far beyond anything I'd ever imagined achieving in my life. But on the morning of the big day my boss in St. Petersburg called the hotel.

"Tree," he said, "I'm sorry to have to do this, but you've got to go to Waco to help out with the Hurricane Katrina victims. Catch the first flight you can get."

"Texas?" I said. "Today? But I'm supposed to make my presentation at one o'clock."

"Sorry, man. They need you there today."

"But … but … can't you get …"

"I know," he said. "It's bad timing, I know. But you're an Environmental Services Manager and that's what they need. We've got to convert an abandoned building into a shelter. By yesterday."

Disappointment and anger immediately engulfed me. "I … I …"

"Nothing I can do about it," he said. "I don't have a reservation for you yet. Maybe you can get a flight out of there after your speech. But you have to go today. Call me back."

I tried to ignore the knot in my stomach as I punched in the airline's phone number. The only seat available on any of the flights to Waco was on a plane that left at 11:00, two hours before I was to speak. I hung my head. Why couldn't they send someone else? It wasn't fair. It was with profound disappointment that I made the airline reservation and called my boss back with the information. He said they'd reserved a room for me at the Ramada Inn and someone would take me there from the airport.

At 1:00 I was looking out the window of the plane to the clouds below, thinking about how well my presentation would have gone, and all the respect and recognition I'd have received. If only … My frustration twisted into anger.

Because of layovers, it was 9 p.m. when I stepped onto the portable steps that had been wheeled out to the plane in Waco. Hot, dry air hit me in the face. I looked around the terminal, which was about the size of two doublewide trailers, and it was clear that no one was there to meet me. I had no idea where to go. After spending the day sitting around in airports waiting for the next flight, my anger was very close to the surface.

I phoned the security station at the Waco V.A., but no one answered. I tried to call my boss back, but couldn't reach him. I asked the cab driver if he knew where I might need to go, but he didn't. All I could think to do was to take a cab to the V.A. Administration Building. When I got there it was 10 p.m. and the place was deserted. Near the end of my rope, I could think of only one thing to do.

I lurked around in the shadows behind the building, where I knew that anyone who saw me would contact security. Sure enough, it wasn't long before a car pulled up with two uniformed men inside. It was an echo from my past. "Can I help you, Buddy?" one of them yelled, sounding a little gruff.

"I hope so," I said, walking to the car. "The Bay Pines V.A. in Florida sent me here to work at a relief center with some of the Katrina survivors, but nobody met me at the airport and I don't know where to go.

"We can help you with that," he said, sounding a lot friendlier. "Get in." It felt strange, sitting in the back seat of a law enforcement vehicle again, but the officers were friendly and drove me to the abandoned three-story building.

Five Naval Public Health workers in starched uniforms were setting up a supply station and triage center to register the survivors as they arrived. Their voices echoed off the bare floors and walls. I introduced myself and they told me I should go to the third floor, where the V.A. command office would be located.

On my way upstairs, I checked out the first two floors. There were no beds or linens, no cooking facilities, office equipment, or cleaning supplies. The only running water was rusty and cold. The building had been empty for three years, and a gray, grimy film covered the walls and floors.

I met several of the other workers and one of them volunteered to take me to the Ramada Inn, where he was also staying. When we arrived, I learned they had no reservation for me and all the rooms were full. The man I was with phoned upstairs and talked to somebody in charge, who called and reserved an entire motel for the use of more workers who were on the way. The fellow took me there and I finally fell into bed, well after midnight.

The next morning at 8:00, the seven of us staying at the motel were taken by shuttle back to our headquarters. After the rest of the management team arrived, we decided to visit the Wal-Mart where one hundred and seventy-five hurricane survivors were being housed. We were told that most had been rescued from rooftops so all their worldly belongings were in the black garbage bags they had with them. This was their third or fourth facility, and like the others, the Wal-Mart had been declared hazardous by the health department. It had to be evacuated as soon as possible.

When we pulled up in front of the building, a few people were standing around outside the door. I said hello as we entered, but they didn't even look up. The next thing that hit me was the revolting stench of garbage and human waste. There were no cooking facilities, showers or washing machines, and the restroom facilities that had been designed for Wal-Mart employees and customers were grossly inadequate for the crowd. There was no way anyone could get clean. Trash bags, mounds of garbage, discarded food, shopping carts, wheelchairs, and walkers surrounded the sleeping mats that covered the filthy floors. Dirty clothes and miscellaneous shoes were everywhere.

On the drive back, the director said, "This is inhumane. We're moving these people tonight." We all agreed it couldn't wait.

At our first full team meeting, the director informed us that the building was being called "The Silver Lining" and our task was to make it operational and friendly to the survivors. Since I was an Environmental Management Service Manager and Hazardous Materials First Responder, I was given the job of contacting the medical center department heads who would help us with supplies, and ensuring that the items were delivered and put to good use.

Instead of just calling the department heads, I decided to meet them in person, hoping that would help keep things running smoothly. I got a ride to the V.A. facility and went from one office to the next, knocking on doors, introducing myself. "Hi, I'm Tree from the Bay Pines V.A. in St. Petersburg, Florida," I said, "and I'm going to be worrying you for the next couple of weeks."

The manager of the laundry area was already in the process of getting washers and dryers installed. The food manager was prepared to start cooking at the facility as soon as they got their supplies in. The warehouse manager agreed to give us temporary cots, hospital beds for those who were ill or disabled, and other furniture we needed. He even gave me a master key to the warehouse so I could get what I needed without having to go through a lot of red tape, and a small Cushman truck to drive to the warehouse and back. The groundskeeper had already dispatched a team to clean up the yard around the facility.

I got back to the Silver Lining around 11 a.m. and we started setting up the rooms. I remembered that the survivors had not had any privacy at all while they were at Wal-Mart, so I spread them out to give them some space to themselves. Families were usually able to have their own rooms, and those requiring electric hospital beds were given private rooms.

When the first bus pulled in we were still placing furniture and moving equipment. I tried to greet everyone, saying, "Welcome. We're glad to have you." Again, not one person answered me. They slumped in line with unkempt hair, ill-fitting clothes, and lost, vacant looks in their eyes. Most walked silently, dragging their black garbage bags. They were directed to a line where they could check in through triage, and while they waited other busloads arrived. At one point the line went along the whole length of the building. Some sat on their bags or on the ground, others leaned against the wall that surrounded the building. Within twenty-four hours we'd moved all the survivors.

Once they cleared triage, they went to the rooms assigned, let their bags fall to the floor and sat down on the cots, waiting to be called for the next meal. When they finished eating, most left the empty Styrofoam containers on the tables in the cafeteria, making no effort to clean up after themselves. Their rooms looked no better. They seemed resigned to a hopeless fate. Life had turned on them. All pride and dignity was absent from their faces. The gravity of enduring so much loss, and having been sent from place to place with no say about where they were to go or how they were to get there, had taken its toll. They seemed to have given up.

The highlight of each day was mealtime, and what survival instincts they seemed to have left became apparent when they got in line early. They'd learned to do that because other shelters had sometimes run out of food.

At first the housekeeping staff complained to me that they shouldn't have to clean up after the adults. "These people didn't need to be waited on hand and foot," they said. "They're not helpless. They're just being lazy."

I reminded them that none of us had lost everything in a devastating flood, and if we had, we might be acting the same way. I encouraged them to keep smiling, just focus on their jobs without being judgmental, and try to keep their comments positive. Grudgingly, they agreed.

While the Public Health staff members were efficient at setting up the triage area, it quickly became clear that several of them were more "job-oriented" than "people-oriented" and did only what was in their orders. They stayed behind their desks and provided information to the survivors and our staff in short, clipped sentences. They often criticized parents whose children were crying or misbehaving and moved off the elevator if more than one or two of the survivors were riding with them. When children ran by, they pulled away, as if they didn't want to be touched.

We had a restricted area for staff use, but there was no signage to let the residents know. When one of the residents wandered in, they said, "You're not allowed in here. Get on back to your area."

When I ran into one of those situations, I kidded the resident, saying something like, "You trying to take my job? Come on, man. I need this job. This back here's just for staff." The next time I picked up supplies in my truck, I got some orange cones and put up a sign. That ended the problem.

Later, one of the housekeepers told me that one of the workers, a Lieutenant Commander in the Navy, insisted that the staff bathroom be cleaned before she entered it each time. I found her sitting at the front desk.

"I'd like to speak to you for a minute," I said.

She gave me a sour look but got up and came into the hall.

"I understand you've asked one of the housekeepers to clean the bathroom before you use it each time."

"That's right," she said, looking me straight in the eye.

"The staff bathroom has a lock on the door. That's the room you're talking about?"

"That's right," she said. "And your point?"

"First, if you have a special request for the housekeeping staff, it needs to go through me. Second, the housekeepers are already overwhelmed with all the work they're doing and cannot possibly do what you're asking and take care of the survivors too."

"Listen," she said, squinting at me. "That bathroom is so filthy that I can't use it without getting my uniform dirty."

"I repeat. The housekeepers will not be doing any special cleaning for you. That bathroom has a lock on it. I suggest you talk to your other staff members about keeping it clean."

She walked away from me without another word, and gave me dirty looks during the rest of her stay. Thankfully, she and her staff were transferred somewhere else a short time later and at that point the V.A. took over the entire facility.

We did our best to get residents to throw away their garbage bags, most of which were contaminated. Many had been soaked in the filthy floodwaters and still held mementos that had been covered with wet, moldy clothing for weeks. Some of the young children's underwear had been soiled but the parents figured they could be washed and bleached at some point down the line. These people had held on to their meager items through flood, rain and rescue, moving from one place to another. How could I tell them that they must give up their only reminders of home? When asked, many refused to give up anything at all, so we provided cleaning supplies and the housekeepers helped them sanitize what they had.

Everyone had been promising them so much for so long that trust was a huge issue. A silver lining actually started to appear, however, when the Red Cross arrived on the fourth day with vouchers for clothing and luggage. Finally they were able to receive financial, physical, and spiritual help. A church organization picked up soiled clothes and returned them washed and folded. Promises that had been made but not kept in other shelters had finally been fulfilled. I started to see a sparkle in the survivors' eyes. A small seed of trust had been planted.

Two days later the first buses arrived to pick the children up to take them to school. Mothers and fathers waited by the front of the building to see their kids off and greeted them in the afternoons.

Now able to bathe, buy clean outfits and wash some of their things, the residents' attitudes changed. We provided transportation to stores and shopping centers and gave advice on purchasing luggage and new toys. Survivors started putting their trash in garbage cans. They straightened up their rooms. Pride and dignity began to return. They started taking charge of their persons, their families and their lives. The seed of trust was starting to flower.

In a room near the elevators there was a woman named Theresa. Every time I passed her and her four children I said, "Good morning," or "Good afternoon," but she never answered. By the fifth day, it occurred to me that she might feel like I was being pushy with her, so I walked by without comment. Just before I turned the corner, I heard her call out, "Hello, Tree." I turned and smiled at her, gave her a wave, and said, "Good morning, Theresa!"

Another of the arrivals was Marcus, a young man taller than my 6'6", who had the mind of a ten-year-old. He'd stand in the hall asking all who went by, "What's your name? Where are you going? Why you doing that?" One day I assigned him the job of hall monitor by the laundry room, and told him he could help me keep track of things. He gave me a huge smile, straightened his shoulders and said, "Yes sir!" Later in the week he was evaluated by our social workers and psychology personnel, and was placed on much needed medication.

A couple who had been planning a wedding decided to go ahead with it, and donations from the staff were used to rent the bride a beautiful wedding dress. The chaplain organized a chorus that sang at the ceremony. Marcus was right there in the middle, singing his heart out, although he didn't know any of the words.

Clarence was an eleven-year-old boy who'd seen his father shot and killed during a burglary, and was left responsible for his mentally challenged mother and physically disabled sister. I saw him with them in the dining hall every day. He always fed his sister before he ate.

An older woman in a wheelchair was deaf and going blind, and for days she wouldn't speak at all. Before we left, she wrote such an endearing letter of thanks that we read it at our closing ceremony. Each staff member received a copy of that letter.

One of the residents gave birth to her third child, a healthy baby boy. I believe the staff, who had been so critical at first, celebrated as much as the family did. Everyone immediately fell in love with him. They even fought over who was going to feed and care for him next. His mother was very happy with all the attention.

Two days before I left, the staff pooled their money and organized a Karaoke party. It was held outside late one afternoon, and the crowd was really into the loud, uplifting music. An old New Orleans blues man sang a song he'd written expressing his gratitude, and Marcus never stopped dancing, with staff members, by himself, and with anyone who came close to him. When kids started break dancing on the grass outside, we tore down some cardboard boxes for them to use to keep from hurting themselves.

I left the party to move some furniture inside, and on a break sat at the top of the outside staircase to the second floor. I looked out at the families and staff. Nurses held babies while children played and their parents danced and talked. Young men danced with elderly ladies using their walkers. Men and women, hopeless ten days before, were laughing and helping each other. The energy changed as people were able to take charge of their lives, make decisions, and plan their next moves.

As I looked out at them, tears started coming. I put on my sunglasses and pretended I had something in my eye, while looking around to make sure nobody saw. A moment later a little boy ran up the stairs and offered me a tissue. He grinned and pointed to his mother, Theresa, the woman who hadn't spoken to me the first few days.

She waved and mouthed the words, "Thank you," a gesture that touched my heart.

The next morning one of the staff engineers found an old trophy in one of the closets and had it engraved with Marcus's name as "Best Dancer." We staged a big staff management meeting the next day and called Marcus in. While he was waiting he kept asking "Why you want me here? What you gonna do? Do I have to move again?"

The ceremony started with the engineer asking Marcus to come forward. He reached out and shook Marcus's hand as he said, "In honor of the energy and quality of dancing that was observed yesterday during Karaoke, Marcus, you were voted 'Best Dancer.'" Marcus stuck his chest out so far I thought he'd strain his back. He grinned from ear to ear and posed as pictures were being snapped. As we congratulated him, Marcus said, "Can I go show my mom?" No sooner had we said yes than he took off, bursting with pride, running down the hall shouting, "Look what I got! Look what I got!" We all wiped the tears away.

I'd come to this job full of anger, feeling I'd been cheated out of a great opportunity. Instead, I got a new respect for life, for people, and for the V.A. Medical Community. I learned firsthand that patience and understanding, along with baths and clean clothes, can begin to build trust and restore dignity. In that small community, a group of dedicated people who forgot their ranks and worked as equals, made the world a better place. Being a part of that experience was far more gratifying than giving a speech could ever have been.

Conclusion

✦

2006

In 2005, Cathy's father died. She talked often about being grateful that she was able to spend time with him after she'd quit drinking. It made me think about the fact that I hadn't seen my own father since I'd been sober, in almost eight years. I'd sent him birthday and holiday cards, and talked to him on the phone, but that was it. I'd always respected my dad, but I'd always feared him, too. Every time I could remember going to see him, it was to ask him for something, usually money, and I'd always been ashamed of myself and of the way I looked.

After hearing Cathy talk about her dad, I decided I needed to go see mine. Just before Christmas 2005 I called Pop and Mama Cleo, and told them I'd like to come for a visit; they said they'd love to see me. Next, I called Puff and Kelsey and they both agreed that they'd like to have me visit. Before I lost my nerve, I made a reservation to fly to Portsmouth for the first weekend in May 2006. That date was so far in the future that I didn't have to worry about it immediately, but since I'd already paid for the airline ticket, I was sure I'd go. I also reserved a rental car and a hotel room that was near my pop's place. That way I wouldn't have to depend on anybody, and if I got into a situation where I wasn't comfortable I'd be able to leave easily.

As May approached, I got more and more anxious about making the trip. Even though they'd all said they wanted me to come, I kept having second thoughts about going back there. I'd been taught that I didn't have to worry about other people's reactions if I just did the next right thing for the next right, good reason. But I still had a hard time letting it all go.

Some years before, Pop had been through a bout with cancer. He'd had his voice box removed, so he talked with a hand-held electronic device. Although his voice sounded mechanical, I could always understand what he was saying when we spoke on the telephone. But I missed hearing his real voice. He'd always been a powerful speaker, and it made me sad to think I'd never hear his voice again.

On the flight up I tried hard not to think about what the next few days might hold. I'd been taught to live in the moment and turn the future over to a higher power, but it wasn't easy.

I checked into the hotel that Friday afternoon and went to see Pop. I was nervous on my way there; my stomach was in knots. I'd long ago paid him back the money I'd borrowed, and I was glad of that. This time I was going to see him because I really wanted to, not because I had to ask him for something or because I owed him something.

It was a beautiful sunny afternoon when I stepped onto that same sidewalk I'd first walked up when I was thirteen years old, all alone and scared to death. As always, the house looked well kept, and there were still flowers in the front yard, but there was a different car in the driveway. I rang the doorbell, and as always, Mama Cleo opened the door.

"Hairston, he's here," she called out, just like she had the first time, forty years before. I smiled at her and she gave me a long, warm hug, then held me at arm's length and said, "You're taller. Or maybe I'm shorter." She laughed and took a step back, "And you cut your hair! You look so nice." She hugged me again. "It's good to see you," she said. "So good to see you."

There was none of the old hesitation in her voice, as there had been years ago. She'd always been supportive, but when I'd shown up before, trouble was always in the air. This time I was welcomed without any reservation.

Instead of leading me back to my father's den as she always had, she took me to the living room, a place used only for very special occasions. My father stood in the doorway, smiling at me. It was the first time I'd ever seen that look on his face. I reached out to shake his hand and he took it, then gave me the first hug he'd ever given me. He put a small metal cylinder to his throat and said in a raspy, electronic voice, "You're okay." It wasn't a question. It was a statement.

We sat down in the living room, me on the sofa with Mama Cleo, and him in a chair.

"How you doing, Pop?" I asked him. "How you feeling?"

"Oh, I'm fine," he said. "Everything's just fine."

I looked over at Mama Cleo and she smiled. "He's doing good. I take good care of him."

Pop asked me, "How have you been?" His face was different, more open. He seemed genuinely interested in what I was going to say. While I talked about my job and life in Florida, I felt like he really listened without looking for something to criticize.

After a pause in the conversation, Mama Cleo stood up. "I'm going to call Calvin," she said, leaving the room. "See what's holding him up."

"Good," I said. "I really want to see him."

She came and went periodically after that, offering food and drinks, then leaving us alone. The smile never left my father's face.

When it was time for the evening news, something my pop never missed, he stood up and motioned for me to follow him back into his den. He sat down in his armchair in front of the TV and flipped it on. I sat in a chair beside him and looked around the familiar room. It still held all his war mementos including pictures of ships he'd served on. On his desk I was pleased to see a picture of Cathy and me that I'd sent a while back. As the newscasters did their work, I soaked up the feel of the room where my father had spent so much of his life.

When the news was over he turned the TV off and I thought to myself, *This is the time for me to start making amends. Now.* At just that point, he turned to me and said, "Billy Junior, I want to tell you that there's one thing I'm sorry about. And that is that I had to learn things about you from the newspaper." He was referring to an article that had appeared Portsmouth's Virginian-Pilot newspaper in October 2005, called "A Family Addiction." A reporter and photographer had come to Florida and spent an entire day with me, hoping to better understand how drug and alcohol abuse affects relatives of the addict.

"Till I read that story, I never knew what happened to you in Vietnam," Pop said. "You never told me. Why?"

"I didn't think you'd believe me," I said. "Nobody else did."

"I wish you'd come to me. I'm ex-military, son. I would have believed you."

I looked down and shook my head. "I wish I had, too," I said.

"I didn't know your life had been so hard."

I leaned forward, my elbows on my knees. With my heart in my throat, I said, "Pop, there are some things I want to say to you." I took a deep breath. "First of all, I'm sorry I didn't take heed to your council, that I never confided in you or really tried to follow your example. You encouraged me to get to know your side of the family and I didn't do that. I wish I'd been able to let you get to know me and that I'd gotten to know you."

Then I sat up straight. "I've always loved and respected you," I said, "but I didn't know how to be a son; or how to be a man. When I started getting clean, I remembered the things you used to tell me. Like the time I came to you to borrow money for a car, and you said, 'You want a car, but you have no place to park it.'"

He nodded.

"When I got out of treatment, I bought my first home, twenty miles away from where I worked. For months, every morning I got up at 4:30 and rode my bike a half-hour to the bus station, then I rode the bus another hour and a half to get to work. But I remembered what you had told me all those years before, and I got my home first."

He looked at me and smiled. Nodding he said, "I knew you could do it."

"And I've just bought myself a really nice condo."

"That's good," he said. "That's real good."

When I heard Calvin come in the front door, I knew we had said all that needed to be said. We returned to the living room and I reached out to shake Calvin's hand. He hugged me and said, "Doggone! Look at that rascal. He done cut his hair."

"Good to see you, man," I said, smiling.

"We're gonna take you to the barbershop, boy. Remember Leroy's Barbershop? His son cuts hair there now. We're gonna get you a professional haircut, now you're a hot-shot manager." We sat down and he said, "Glad you're here, man. We're so glad you're here."

After Mama Cleo served us a great supper, we sat in the living room and talked about friends and relatives, the changes in the world, and the war in Iraq. For the first time in my entire life, I actually felt like I was a part of my family.

When I got back to the hotel, I called the AA Central Office and learned there was a meeting just down the street. It was exactly what I needed.

Driving back to my hotel after the meeting, tears came to my eyes as I thought of the day gone by, of the smile on my father's face. Tonight I'd seen a different man from the one I'd always known. Tonight, he was my father. It took me a long time to stop crying.

When I woke the next morning, I was really nervous about seeing my daughters. I reminded myself that they had wanted to see me, and that everything would be all right.

I had breakfast with Pop, Mama Cleo, and Calvin; and then Calvin took me for the "professional" haircut he'd promised. Leroy's Barbershop was the same as it had been forty years before, full of old men hanging out there half the day talking baseball and politics.

Then I went to see Kelsey and her husband, Joe in their large new home. She had told me that they'd be holding a party that night in honor of Bett's birthday and invited me to come. Although I wasn't looking forward to seeing Bett, I agreed.

Kelsey and Joe's two boys were five and seven, handsome young men. They welcomed me into the living room and Kelsey brought in some cookies to eat while we talked; Joe and the boys seemed comfortable with me, but there was a definite tension with Kelsey. She kept getting up and going into the kitchen, saying she was getting things ready for the afternoon barbecue. When she decided that they needed more food, she made up a list and Joe and I went to the store. When we got back, friends and relatives had started arriving and were drinking, talking and laughing as they watched sports on the two large-screen TVs. The party was underway. The kind of party I'd attended so many times in my life.

I said hello to old friends and talked for a while, then went to find Kelsey. She was in the kitchen alone, washing dishes. The room was filled with plates of food others had brought, a big pot of mashed potatoes, gravy, a huge tray of chicken ready to barbeque, along with bowls of vegetables, garlic bread, salad, coolers of beer and bottles of liquor. I said, "Um, Kelsey, I have a few things I'd like to say to you."

She glanced up as she continued working, "Okay."

I took a deep breath and leaned back against the sink. "I know I wasn't a good father to you and Puff. In fact, I sucked at it. I was unsupportive and irresponsible, and I used drugs as an excuse. But there was no excuse for what I did."

Kelsey glanced up at me as she scrubbed a pot, hard.

"I'm grateful that you've turned out so well," I said. "You were always dependable, so loving." I paused but she didn't say anything, just kept scrubbing. "I wish I could change the past, God knows, I wish I could."

Her scrubbing slowed.

"There is something I *can* do, though. I love you, Kelsey, and from now on, I want to be there for you. From this day forward."

She rinsed the pot silently, put it in the dish drainer, and turned off the water. "I've been mad at you since you moved to Florida," she said. "It felt like you didn't want to be with us. Like you didn't care about us."

"I'm sorry."

"And when we brought the kids down to Disney World, you didn't even come over to see them. That wasn't right."

"I really wanted to see you. I wish it could have been different," I said. "I truly do."

She dried her hands on a towel and turned to face me, leaning back against the counter. "I've been learning a lot about alcoholism lately. And I do understand Mom better. Addiction is an awful thing isn't it?"

"Yes. It is."

She paused and looked down. "You know, maybe moving to Florida *was* the best thing for you to do. I still don't like the fact that you left us, but maybe you had to do that to get sober. Maybe that helped you sink down so low that you finally hit your bottom."

"Maybe so."

"They say that's the only way alcoholics can ever give up the drink."

"That's right."

She looked at me. "I really want to do the right thing for Mama," she said, "but I just can't see her so unhappy and not help out. I can't let her hit bottom."

"That's the only way she's gonna get better," I said.

"I don't think I can do that," she said. "But I'm glad it worked for you. It shows."

She walked toward my open arms and I hugged my daughter. I couldn't remember the last time I'd hugged her, and it felt wonderful. "I love you," I said.

"I love you, too, Daddy," she said in a trembling voice.

Later that evening Puff phoned the house to talk to me, saying she was sorry she hadn't been able to come to the party. Even though I wasn't able to see her, I was able to talk to her as I had to Kelsey. I said that I knew I hadn't been there for her and her sister years ago, and that I want to be a better father to them in the future.

With both of my girls, when I felt they wanted to stop talking about the past, I did.

Bett arrived at the party a little late, but all dressed up for her birthday. She came over and hugged me and it felt strange to me to be in the same room with the woman who had been my wife for so many years. She looked much the same, just older, and she sounded the same. We talked a little, but it felt awkward and she soon went off to get something to drink.

After we'd eaten all the barbecue, an ice cream truck came by and I bought a treat for each of the kids; by that time, there must have been forty of them. The guy driving the truck told me he remembered me from elementary school, and although I couldn't quite place him, he gave me a discount.

When it was time to leave, I said my goodbyes to everyone but Bett. She'd fallen asleep in a chair, as she had done so many times in years past. It reinforced to me that I was where I was supposed to be.

My sister Ivy was the only one I hadn't seen, so I drove to the small apartment she had just moved into. She was in bed when I arrived, but got up and gave me a hug. She apologized for the condition of the place and we talked for a few minutes but I could see that she felt uncomfortable with me. It was clear that she'd been going through hard times, so before I left I gave her some money. I told her I hoped to spend more time with her when I came to visit again.

The next morning, I went to church with Mama Cleo, Calvin, and his daughter. The pastor asked Mama Cleo to introduce me, and I stood up beside her. "I want everybody to meet my son, Tree," she said.

"He's your son, is that right?" the pastor asked.

"Yes, sir. He's my son," she said proudly, giving me a big smile. When we sat down she patted my arm and gave it a squeeze.

The family knew that I had to leave before the service was over to catch my plane and when the time came, I got up and tried to sneak out quietly, in part to hide my tears. But they followed me and hugged me goodbye on the steps of the church. I was overwhelmed by the love I felt. I truly was a part of my family.

As my plane came in for a landing in Tampa, I thought about how glad I was to have gone back to Portsmouth; how facing my past puts me one step closer to becoming the man I've always wanted to be.

I thanked my higher power for my new life in sobriety.

And I recognized how very good it was to be back home.